ENJOY SMART SUGARS

YOUR SUPPORT GUIDE

Multiple research studies conclude that certain sugars improve brain function.

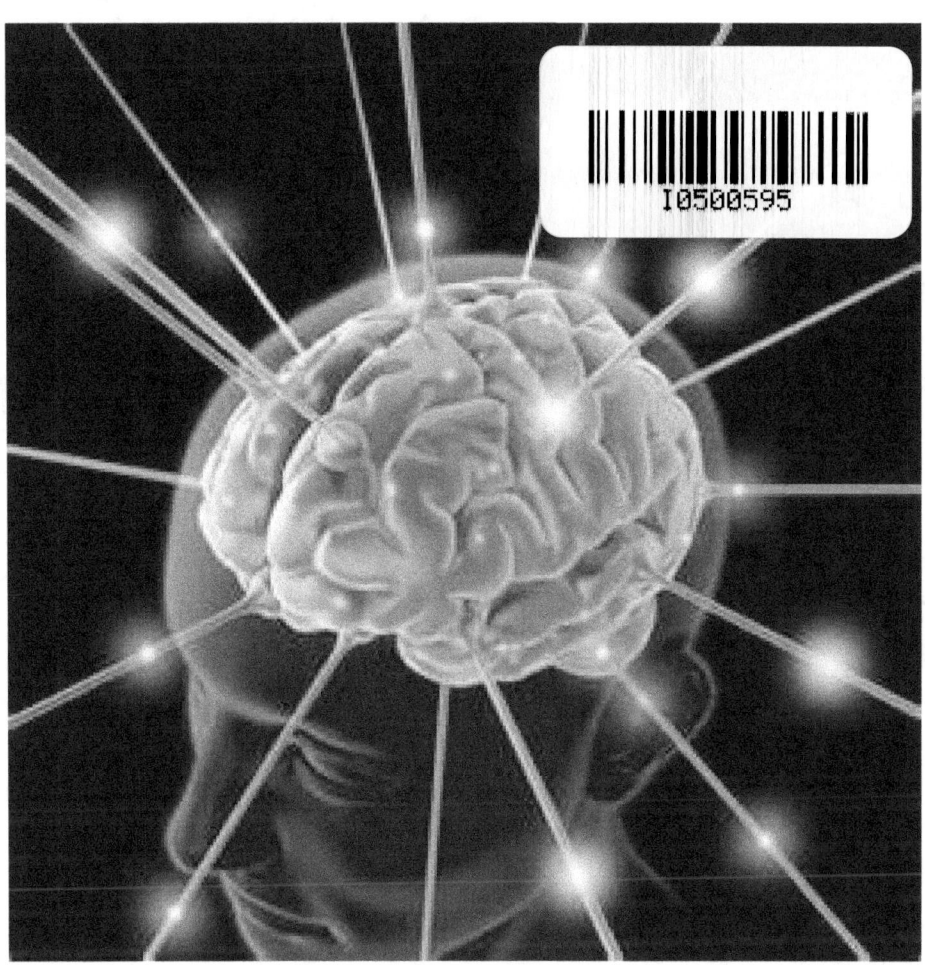

This book is your guide to help you improve brain function, overcome stress, become healthier, and advance medical science.

Learn if you qualify to participate in a Pilot Survey and we welcome your doctor to observe.

INCLUDES GLYCOSCIENCE LESSONS SUPPORTING PILOT STUDIES

This is not a booklet of ideas. This is an ACTION book and the next step is up to you.

JC SPENCER

AN EDUCATIONAL PROJECT OF

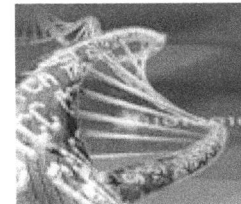

THE ENDOWMENT FOR MEDICAL RESEARCH

Your Source For News and Education In Glycomics The Science of Sugars

Contents of this booklet are informational.
No medical claims are made or intended.

ISBN-13: 978-1482779813
ISBN-10: 1482779811

Introduction to Enjoy Smart Sugars
Y O U R   S U P P O R T   G U I D E

The new frontier of medical science is the ultrahigh-technology breakthrough in the branch of biology called Glycobiology or Glycoscience. (Glyco is Greek for sugar). Indeed, Glycoscience is the future of medicine. Glycoscience is now proven to be the bull's eye, the Rosetta Stone, the Holy Grail of medicine and of all healthcare. MIT is on record of saying that Glycoscience will change the way we live.

Smart Sugars will become more widely known to the general public and healthcare professionals. Their extreme beneficial properties for good health will become understood as Glycoscience education is made available.

Glycoscience makes for good communication.
Good communication makes everything happen.

Smart Sugars actually are the building blocks of the Operating System (OS) of the human body that processes all communication within the body. The OS reads, translates, and transcribes the DNA for every cell in your body. Corrupted glycans and glycoproteins alter gene expression and result in disease and death. Communication makes everything happen. Mis-communication makes things happen wrong. This is the beginning of understanding Glycoscience.

Doctors of tomorrow will better understand Glycoscience than today's generation. **Transforming Glycoscience** (the work prepared by the National Research Council of the National Academies) recommends that all universities and high schools Glycoscience.

Every significant scientific organization and association went on record in 2012 that: **"*Glycans impact the structure/function of every living cell in humans, animals, and plants.*"** A panel was appointed from The National Academies: The National Research Council, National Academy of Science, the National Academy of Engineering, the Institute of Medicine, the National Research Council, the National Institutes of Health, National Science Foundation, and the Food and Drug Administration to write **Transforming Glycoscience - A Roadmap for the Future.**

Glycoscience is the future of medicine and healthcare and will forever change our medical system. Traditional medicine through pharmaceutical companies will synthesize various Smart Sugars to make new drugs. The new drugs, using a piece of Glycoscience technology, will indeed work better and be less toxic. Other new glyco drugs will help develop superior immunology breakthroughs. But, there is a better way. Integrating natural specific Smart Sugar into your daily consumption of food will increase glycosylation of cells to produce more stem cells which are designed to maintain and repair. Glycoscience reintroduces the values of the Father of Medicine, Hippocrates, who said, **"*Let food be thy medicine and medicine be thy food.*"**

Table of Contents

Section One - Educational Materials

Section Two - Research

Section Three - Trehalose, One Smart Sugar

Section Four - Find Out More with Online Resources

Section Five - Test Your Brain Games

Section Six - Forms for Action

Glycoscience Education

Education for tomorrow's doctors, healthcare professionals, and general public about the New Frontier of Medicine. The basic knowledge of Glycoscience is summarized in the authoritative whitepaper. This publication is available online as an interactive magazine and can be downloaded at http://Glycosciencewhitepaper.com and is available in 100 pound quality glossy stock for training purpose. Educators are using the Glycoscience whitepaper to teach their students.

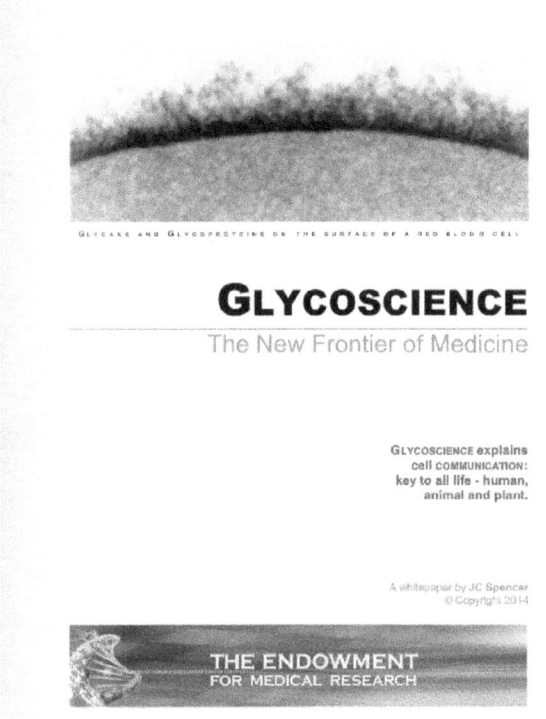

GLYCANS AND GLYCOPROTEINS ON THE SURFACE OF A RED BLOOD CELL

GLYCOSCIENCE
The New Frontier of Medicine

GLYCOSCIENCE explains
cell COMMUNICATION:
key to all life - human,
animal and plant.

A whitepaper by JC Spencer
© Copyright 2014

THE ENDOWMENT
FOR MEDICAL RESEARCH

The authoritative Glycoscience whitepaper

Professors, Physicians, Healthcare Professionals and the General Public are welcome to use the online interactive whitepaper without charge.

http://Glycosciencewhitepaper.com

Educators use the whitepaper to train their students.

The Glycoscience whitepaper is also available from http://GlycoscienceBooks.com

Advance Glycoscience Training is available

14 hours Professional Glycomics DVD Training Series from our First Glycomics Medical Conference for Healthcare Professionals includes 500 page syllabus of all the color slides presented (Regular price for this quality education with CME/CEU Credits is $1,995.) Note: Credits have expired - Sales price for limited time is only $199.

14 hours General Public Glycomics DVD Training Series for the General Public (does not include 500 page syllabus of all the color slides presented.) Sales price for limited time is only $99   Orders may be made online at http://GlycoscienceBooks.com

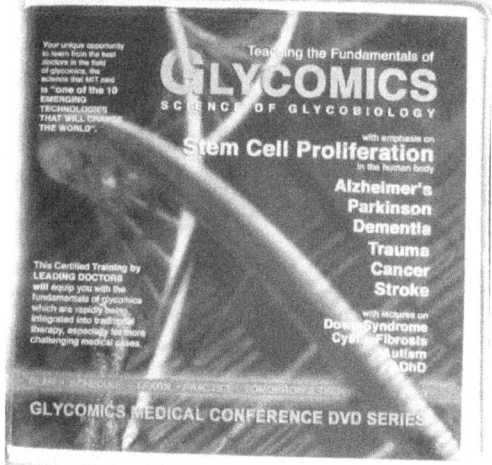

Stem Cell Survey - A Technical Syllabus on CD by H. Reg McDaniel, MD provided for use by Healthcare Professionals. Evidence that Glycomics can increase stem cell proliferation and stem cell function in humans. Learning and Behavior Problems in Children Responsive to Micronutrients Led to Benefits Reported in Infants and Youth and Maternal Alcohol Damage (FAS). Your contribution of $50 serves as a fundraiser and is shared between The Endowment for Medical Research and the Fisher Institute for Medical Research.

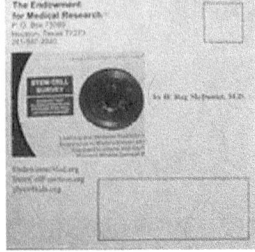

Additional reading and training materials
FREE online support continuing
Glycomicscience Education and Research.

Readers have access to hundreds of hours of FREE online
materials in the form of articles, reports, and video clips.
This is a part of the educational effort of
The Endowment for Medical Research, Inc.

http://endowmentmed.org

http://Glycosciencewhitepaper.com

http://GlycoscienceNEWS.com

http://DiabeticHope.com

Details on booking JC Spencer for lectures at universities, organizations, and fund raising events contact him at jcs@endowmentmed.org or 281-587-2020

Smart Sugars is *NOW* available in
Hardbound, Soft cover, Kindle and in Audio

Available world wide on Amazon or in our
Bookstore: http://GlycoscienceBooks.com

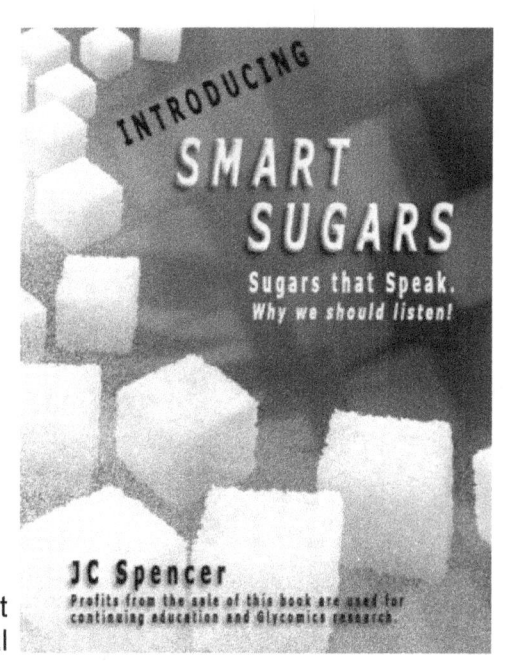

Read this book and learn
WHY WE SHOULD LISTEN!

Introducing Smart Sugars -
Sugars that Speak. Why we should listen!

An introduction to Glycoscience. Easy to read for the student while packed with new information for the seasoned medical professional, research scientist, and learned professor.

Now available in audio on Amazon   (play audio sample) (cut & paste Link)
http://audible.com.au/pd/Health-Personal-Development/Smart-Sugars-Audiobook/B00OGNKFCA

Go to http://Amazon.com and type in Smart Sugars to see what is available.
Click on the authors name for other Glycoscience related books.

Smart Sugars [Unabridged]
Audible Audio Edition

by JC Spencer (Author) with Ross Merrick (Narrator)

Listen on your Kindle Fire or with the free Audible app on Apple, Android, and Windows devices.

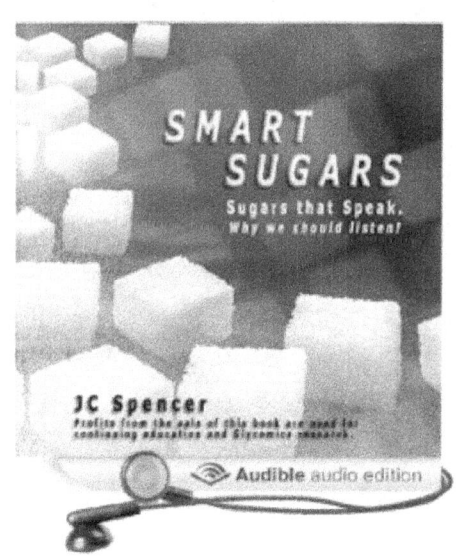

Order online after you listen to a audio sample
of the reading of Smart Sugars
http://SmartSugars.com/audio or

http://amazon.com/Smart-Sugars/dp/B00OI2H6VW/ref=sr_1_sc_1?ie=UTF8&qid=
1414528141&sr=8-1-spell&keywords=Smart+Surgars+audio+book

Read the Editorial Reviews on Amazon

Smart Sugars is an easy to read book about the breakthrough of sugar technology that will change the way we live. The author explains that some 800,000 transmitting antennae called glycans (actually sugar) coat each of our healthy cells like fuzz on a peach. **Smart Sugars** will help us take the focus off of the disease, treat and cure, because of these new discoveries. Tomorrow's doctors will use Glycoscience diagnostics to read our cells to better determine health and what our health will or can be years in advance.

This Glycoscience textbook is for the inquisitive individual and the learned scientist.

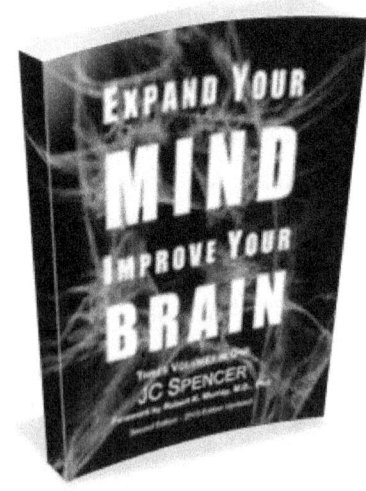

Expand Your MIND
Improve Your BRAIN

is an easy to read entertaining 580 page science book that references over 700 MDs, PhDs, Scientists, Researchers and Educators in the field of Glycomicscience and Brain Function.

Available Three Volumes in One or
Volumes One, Two, and Three Separately.

Updated in 2016
Available in e-textbook,
perfect bound 8 1/5 x 11,
and hardbound editions.

First Edition published
in 2008 - Second Edition
published 2013

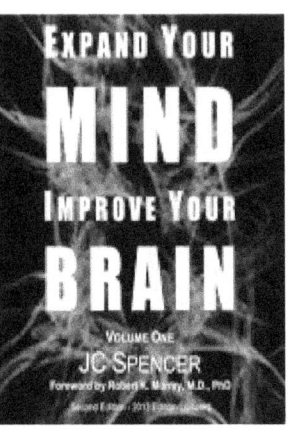 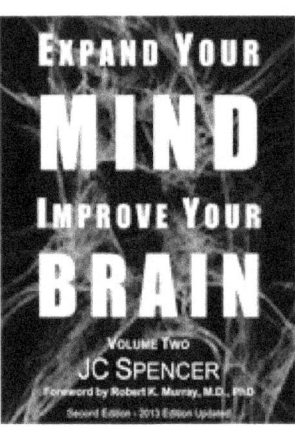 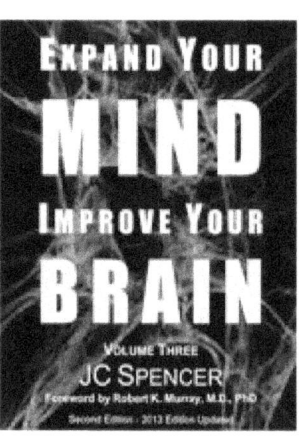

Three Volumes in One
    Softbound .... $ 77.77
    Hardbound $127.77

Vol. 1; Vol. 2; and Vol. 3 available individually as an ebook ..... $ 27.77 each
Three Volumes in One e-textbook .... $ 47.77

Glycoscience 101

presents 101 Glycoscience Lessons.
The author explains how Glycoscience
is the New Frontier of Medicine.
And, how Glycoscience education
will equipt tomorrow's doctors.

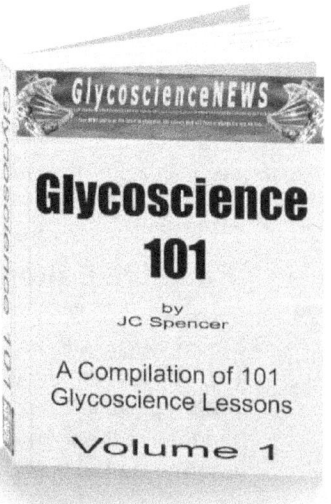

The Trehalose Handbooks are available Three Volumes in One or Volume One, Two, and Three Separately.

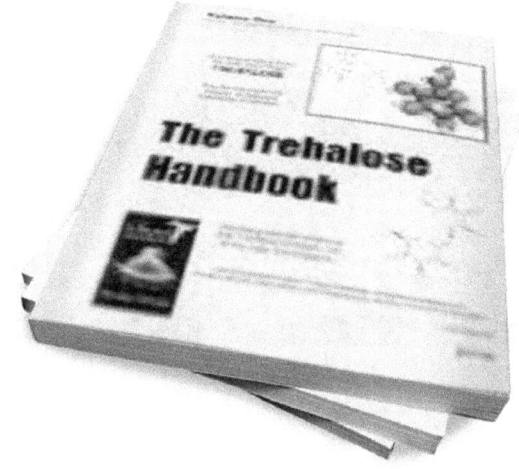
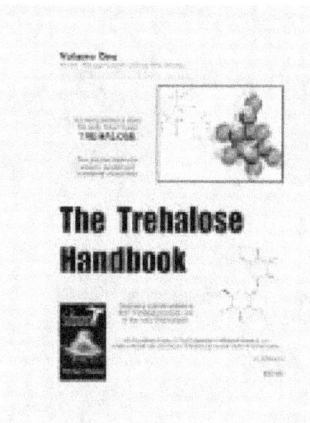
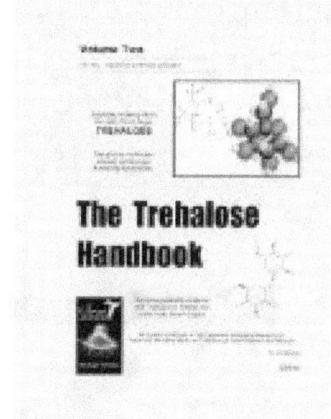

Available on Amazon and in the Glycoscience Book Store at
http://GlycoscienceBooks.com

Ebola Lies

Learn HOW Ebola and other viruses can take charge of the human body. Also, learn about the Glycan / Glycoprotein connection to viruses.

2.1

Exposing Lies with Documented Truth and How You Can Protect Yourself and Your Loved Ones

Updated in 2016 with a chapter about how the Zika virus endangers the human race even more than Ebola.

by JC Spencer

WHY EBOLA BECAME POLITICAL!

WARNING: Do NOT read this book unless you are open to verifiable truth that is disturbing.

The book solves the Zika mystery of HOW the mosquito became so harmful by altering the DNA to cause birth defects to form small brains in human babies.

Available world-wide on Amazon or from
http://GlycoscienceBooks.com

Ebola is designed to kill millions!

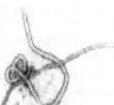

Ebola can cross the oceans in a single bound, just a plane flight away. The bubonic plague bacteria killed millions in years gone by. Ebola is a serial killer.

Ebola caught humans ill prepared. Politicians disconnected from medical reality may do more harm than good as the embers of the most infectious epidemic smolder under cover of deception.

In a frontal attack on the immune system, Ebola gains a beachhead for victory over humans. With amazing military skill Ebola sets aside the generals of the white blood cell army. It goes straight for the kill by transmitting a message for the cells to surrender their glycoprotein defense system. Within a few days, the human is conquered as structured glycoproteins are fractured into non-structured glycoproteins. These non-structured glycoprotein snippets become the decoys that further confuse the remaining defenders of the immune system.

Billions of dollars are flung at developing new drugs. But, the real answer lies in equipping the existing army of the immune system. Only about 10% of us have an immune system that can kill Ebola. Learn life saving instructions in Ebola Lies.

Some enemies are subtle and some are not so subtle. The purpose we all have is to protect our families from all enemies foreign and domestic. The purpose of Ebola Lies is to enable the reader to help save lives and improve individual health. Anything that endangers your life must be exposed and correction.

What you don't know can kill you!

Ebola Lies answers questions the media are not asking and supports the answers with documented evidence.

Ebola Lies separates FACTS from MYTHS.

The NEWS: People are thinking about what is the HEALTHIEST SUGAR. But, few understand what is healthy or sugar. The Huffington Post presented this sugar graph which reveals how confusing is the issue.

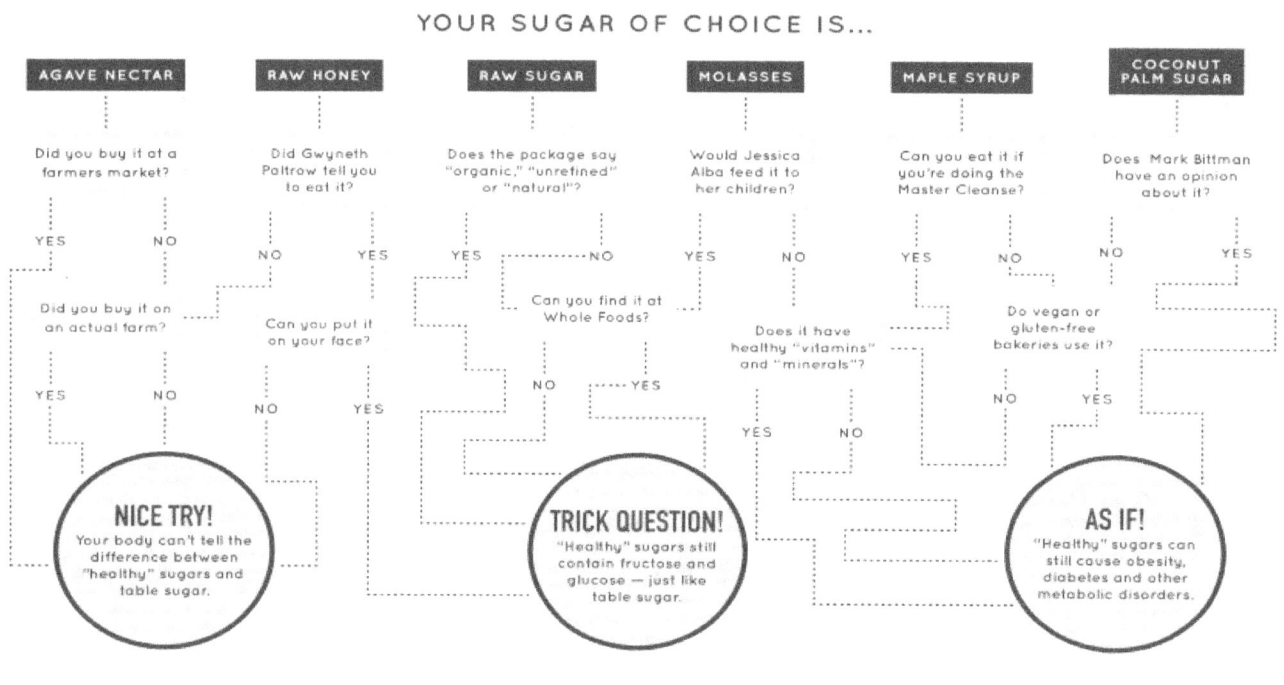

All three circles above, NICE TRY!, TRICK QUESTION!, and AS IF! are ..... __ALL WRONG!__

Your body knows the difference between good and bad sugars. Every harmful and every beneficial sugar is unique and has a different biological function. Some Smart Sugars are beneficial to put on your face! Skin care companies have recently added Trehalose to their formulas. Trehalose is now in the skin care products of Estée Laider, L'Oréal, MAX Factor, Revlon, Avon, and Merl Norman to mention a few.

Glycoscience is changing the way we live. Education of the reality of Smart Sugars will enable us to benefit today by applying this advanced technology discovered from decades of research. The Endowment for Medical Research and the GlycoScience Institute are committed to educate the world about Glycoscience. We will make available the benefits or harm each sugar and sweetener has on the human body.

Major Glycoscience Research in Obesity, Depression, Neurological Challenges and Diabetes

NEW Research indicates Trehalose may inhibit Fatty Liver

Sci. Signal. 23 Feb 2016:
Vol. 9, Issue 416, pp. ra21
DOI: 10.1126/scisignal.aac5472

Trehalose inhibits solute carrier 2A (SLC2A) proteins to induce autophagy and prevent hepatic steatosis, Brian J. DeBosch, Monique R. Heitmeier, Allyson L. Mayer, Cassandra B. Higgins, Jan R. Crowley, Thomas E. Kraft, Maggie Chi, Elizabeth P. Newberry, Zhouji Chen, Brian N. Finck, Nicholas O. Davidson, Kevin E. Yarasheski, Paul W. Hruz, and Kelle H. Moley, *Sci. Signal.* 2016, **9**, ra21 DOI: 10.1126/scisignal.aac5472

Trehalose is a naturally occurring disaccharide that has gained attention for its ability to induce cellular autophagy and mitigate diseases related to pathological protein aggregation. Despite decades of ubiquitous use as a nutraceutical, preservative, and humectant, its mechanism of action remains elusive. We showed that trehalose inhibited members of the SLC2A (also known as GLUT) family of glucose transporters. Trehalose-mediated inhibition of glucose transport induced AMPK (adenosine 5'-monophosphate–activated protein kinase)–dependent autophagy and regression of hepatic steatosis in vivo and a reduction in the accumulation of lipid droplets in primary murine hepatocyte cultures. Our data indicated that trehalose triggers beneficial cellular autophagy by inhibiting glucose transport.

Trehalose Sugar Impacts Growth of Baby Chicks

Research shows that Trehalose may improve natural intestinal immunity in baby chicks

by JC Spencer

How can the sugar Trehalose help weight gain in baby chicks, fat loss in obese men, and lower fats in the liver?

A study published in *British Poultry Science* 2016 March 17 may inch us toward solving the mystery.

In previous Lessons, we have learned how fat cells in obese men are positively affected by Trehalose and the important role that glycolipids play as signaling molecules inside the cell.

Lipids (as high triglycerides) block glucose and fat conversion to energy. However, when certain sugar building blocks are added, glycolipids help transfer glucose and fats through the liver. This results in a healthier liver, superior body functions, and health.

Now comes fascinating research from Tohoku University that indicates Trehalose effects significant growth performance of baby chicks while there was no observed increase in the levels of lipid peroxidation in skeletal muscle, liver, and plasma. Increasing growth while not increasing oxidation of lipids is important because it leads to healthier lean tissue.

It appears to me that lipid peroxidation may be the tipping point for many diseases especially in infants as free radicals damage membrane lipids and eventually tissue. This chain-reaction may implicate many diseases, especially neurological diseases.

Abstract as published: Br Poult Sci. 2016 Mar 17. [Epub ahead of print]

Effects of trehalose supplementation on the growth performance and intestinal innate immunity of juvenile chicks.

Kikusato M[1], Nanto F[1], Mukai K[2], Toyomizu M[1].

1. Trehalose is composed of two molecules of D-glucose joined by an α,α-1,1 glucosidic linkage, and has antioxidative and anti-inflammatory effects. The present study investigated the effect of feeding a trehalose-supplemented diet on the growth performance, as well as the oxidative status and the intestinal innate immunity of juvenile chicks. 2. A total of 24 d-old male broiler chicks were used in this study: two groups of 8 birds were fed on a 0% (control) or 0.5% trehalose-supplemented diet for 18 d. 3. The mean body weight of the trehalose group was significantly greater than that of the control group, but feed efficiency was not altered by feeding the trehalose-supplemented diet. No differences in the levels of lipid peroxidation in skeletal muscle, liver and plasma were observed between the control and trehalose-supplemented groups. The mRNA levels of interferon-γ, tumour necrosis factor-like ligand 1A, interleukin-10, NADPH oxidase 4 and inducible NO synthase were significantly reduced by the trehalose supplementation. 4. Our results suggest that dietary supplementation with trehalose after hatching may have beneficial effects on the growth performance of juvenile chicks, probably by improving their intestinal innate immunity.

(End of Abstract)

Tomorrow's doctors will better understand Glycoscience. Glycoscience is the future of medicine and healthcare.

Source and References:

Animal Nutrition, Life Sciences, Graduate School of Agricultural Science, Tohoku University, 1-1 Tsutsumidori-Amamiyamachi, Sendai, Japan 981-8555.
http://www.ncbi.nlm.nih.gov/pubmed/26986698
Trehalose may lower triglycerides: Abstract
www.ncbi.nlm.nih.gov/pubmed/21147367
www.naturalnews.com/021808_cancer_prevention.html#ixzz3wsjkckwr
Smart Sugars and Your Triglyceride Battle by JC Spencer August 2012
Study Obese men and Trehalose
http://www.endowmentmed.org/content/view/951/33/
http://www.ncbi.nlm.nih.gov/pubmed/?term=Trehalose+obese+men
Expand Your Mind - Improve Your Brain
http://www.endowmentmed.org/content/view/826/106/
Change Your Sugar, Change Your Life
http://DiabeticHope.com

Glycoscience Lesson #40
http://www.GlycoscienceNEWS.com/pdf/Lesson40.pdf
http://EzineArticles.com/?expert=JC_Spencer

Trehalose Anti-Depressant Study
Research indicates that the Smart Sugar Trehalose has an anti-depressant effect. This discovery may open a new pathway for overcoming stress.

JC Spencer, CEO of The Endowment for Medical Research in Houston, Texas, said, "*A newly published paper from Israel shows that Trehalose induced an anti-depressant effect in laboratory animals.*" Mr. Spencer has assisted universities and research laboratories in several countries by supplying the sugar Trehalose to further research.

Professor Haim Einat, Ph.D., with the School of Behavioral Sciences, Tel Aviv-Yaffo Academic College, Tel-Aviv, Israel, one of the authors of the paper, told Mr. Spencer, "*We are continuing to work on the behavioral and biochemical effects of trehalose and we believe that it might have much potential in our field of affective disorders, both as a possible treatment option and as an additional avenue for us to better understand that pathophysiology and treatment mechanisms in depression. I wish to thank you again for you generous donation of trehalose.*"

The collaborative effort included Ben-Gurion University in Beersheba, Israel and the College of Pharmacy, University of Minnesota in Duluth, USA.

The study was designed to explore antidepressant and mood stabilizing activity of trehalose in animal models for depression and mania. It is hypothesized that these behavioral changes could be related to trehalose effects to enhance autophagy. Autophagy is a major protein degradation pathway that is essential for stress-induced and constitutive protein folding. Autophagy is the controlled digestion of damaged organelles within a cell and the maintenance of bodily nutrition by the metabolic breakdown of some bodily tissues. It is necessary for the clearance of toxic protein waste especially from neurons. It is believed that to achieve autophagy enhancement is a significant discovery, especially if further studies confirm that indeed trehalose can play a role in human behavioral levels.

Trehalose has long been known for cell membrane protection against stress, health benefits by helping to properly fold proteins, and is effective against neurodegenerative challenges. This study helps explain the pathway these benefits are accomplished.

The Endowment for Medical Research, a 501 c 3 non-profit research and educational public charity, offers continuing education in the field of glycoscience. A part of their educational program is to make available to the general public free information through http://DiabeticHope.com

The paper was accepted for publication in the journal Psychopharmacology.
The PubMed abstract link is:
http://ncbi.nlm.nih.gov/pubmed/23644913

Trehalose delays the progression of amyotrophic lateral sclerosis by enhancing autophagy in motoneurons.

Castillo K, Nassif M, Valenzuela V, Rojas F, Matus S, Mercado G, Court FA, van Zundert B, Hetz C.

Source
Biomedical Neuroscience Institute; Faculty of Medicine; University of Chile; Santiago, Chile; Center for Molecular Studies of the Cell; Program of Cellular and Molecular Biology; Institute of Biomedical Sciences; University of Chile; Santiago, Chile.

Abstract
Amyotrophic lateral sclerosis (ALS) is a fatal motoneuron disease with no current effective treatment. Accumulation of abnormal protein inclusions containing SOD1, TARDBP, FUS, among other proteins, is a pathological hallmark of ALS. Autophagy is the major degradation pathway involved in the clearance of damaged organelles and protein aggregates. Although autophagy has been shown to efficiently degrade ALS-linked mutant protein in cell culture models, several studies suggest that autophagy impairment may also contribute to disease pathogenesis. In this report, we tested the potential use of trehalose, a disaccharide that induces MTOR-independent autophagy, in the development of experimental ALS. Administration of trehalose to mutant SOD1 transgenic mice significantly prolonged life span and attenuated the progression of disease signs. These effects were associated with decreased accumulation of SOD1 aggregates and enhanced motoneuron survival. The protective effects of trehalose were associated with increased autophagy levels in motoneurons. Cell culture experiments demonstrated that trehalose led to mutant SOD1 degradation by autophagy in NSC34 motoneuron cells and also protected primary motoneurons against the toxicity of conditioned media from mutant SOD1 transgenic astrocytes. At the mechanistic level, trehalose treatment led to a significant upregulation in the expression of key autophagy-related genes at the mRNA level including Lc3, Becn1, Sqstm1 and Atg5. Consistent with these changes, trehalose administration enhanced the nuclear translocation of FOXO1, an important transcription factor involved in the activation of autophagy in neurons. This study suggests a potential use of trehalose and enhancers of MTOR-independent autophagy for the treatment of ALS.

http://ncbi.nlm.nih.gov/pubmed/23851366

Published September 2013

Research Shows: High Triglycerides CAUSE Fat Gain
High Fructose Corn Syrup Produces High Triglycerides
Trehalose Sugar Reduces Triglycerides - HFCS is High Risk and Table Sugar is Also Risk

by JC Spencer

Key to Fat Loss - Triglycerides

Fat loss is impossible when high triglycerides (lipids) block glucose and fat conversion to energy. The primary biological function of these fatty structural molecules is to store and transport fat. When certain sugars are added, the building blocks form glycolipids to become important signaling molecules inside the cell. These non-protein molecules make up the cell and cell membrane that help transfer glucose and fat through the liver.

Overweight people can experience serious fat loss when triglycerides are normal, kept under 150 mg/dL. Over 200 is high and 500 is very high. A healthy lifestyle of good food and proper exercise will inch you closer to your objective.

High triglycerides produce
LDL cholesterol

LDL triggers pancreatic and cardiovascular problems. Studies evidence that statin drugs, prescribed to lower cholesterol, cause even more serious health problems.

How well the carbohydrates we consume will metabolize into glucose and ATP (adenosine triphosphate) is of paramount importance. Evidence from Rutgers University suggests that sodas sweetened with high fructose corn syrup (HFCS) may increase the risk of diabetes and obesity, particularly in children. These drinks and foods laced with HFCS are converted into triglycerides and are stored in the adipose tissue, or fat cells.

Raging Battle Between
the Good, the Bad and the Ugly

The raging fat battle is between good fats and bad fats, good sugars and bad sugars - good and bad carbohydrates. Saturated fats (bad fat) along with bad sugars, especially HFCS, result in high plasma levels of triglyceride-rich lipoproteins which produce glucose intolerance leading to diabetes.

Polyunsaturated fat, (the good fat) as Omega-3, has been shown to lower triglycerides by balancing blood sugar, reducing inflammation, and helping to regulate metabolism. Exactly how this happens is not yet clear, but we understand that Omega-3 decreases lipid synthesis (lipogenesis) and may allow the hormone leptin to work better. Researchers have linked leptin to the process of how fast fat is burned. Leptin is the protein circulated in the bloodstream that goes to the brain which controls how much fat to store in the cells.

The Sugar that Sustains Glucose Levels

One Diabetic/Trehalose study concluded that nano-particles of Trehalose result in sustained release of insulin that causes prolonged reduction of blood glucose levels in diabetic rats.

Research confirms that the sugar Trehalose can inhibit fat cell hypertrophy (cell enlargement) and prevent metabolic syndrome which induces insulin resistance which leads to type 2 diabetes. Findings further suggest Trehalose is a functional saccharide that mitigates insulin resistance resulting in a better sugar balance.

A clinical research paper from a randomized, double-blind, crossover study was designed to assess the effects of Trehalose. The study shows that Trehalose actually helps balance the insulin and glucose concentrations in obese men. This is very important for fat loss.

It is a significant finding that Trehalose elicits lower glycemic and insulinemic responses in obese men as compared with glucose alone.

Source and References:

Trehalose may lower triglycerides: Abstract
http://ncbi.nlm.nih.gov/pubmed/21147367

Smart Sugars and Your Triglyceride Battle by JC Spencer August 2012
Study Obese men and Trehalose
http://endowmentmed.org/content/view/951/33/

http://ncbi.nlm.nih.gov/pubmed/?term=Trehalose+obese+men

Expand Your Mind - Improve Your Brain
http://endowmentmed.org/content/view/826/106/

Change Your Sugar, Change Your Life
http://DiabeticHope.com

Reference: Smart Sugars Lesson #64
http://endowmentmed.org/pdf/SmartLesson64

Reprint: **Glycoscience Lesson #35**
http://GlycoscienceNEWS.com/pdf/Lesson35.pdf

http://EzineArticles.com/?expert=JC_Spencer

Glycoscience - the Study of Sugars

Of the many sugars found in nature only a few are what
I call Smart Sugars. Trehalose is **One Smart Sugar**.

Trehalose Q & A

Trehalose is the sugar everyone would use if they only knew...[TM]
Trehalose LEAVES A FRESH CLEAN TASTE IN YOUR MOUTH...[TM]

Q: What is Trehalose?
A: Trehalose is a sweet healthful sugar. It is two pure glucose molecules bonded uniquely that gives it special functionality. Unlike other sweeteners, Trehalose has amazing ability to improve cells in the human body.

Q: Trehalose is made from what?
A: Trehalose is found in nature and can be produced from tapioca or other starches.

Q: Is Trehalose genetically modified?
A: Purity is important to us. Some Trehalose on the market is imported from China. We do not import from China and our Trehalose is Certified GM Free:

Q: How is Trehalose beneficial?
A: Trehalose is known to strengthen cell membrane and aid the body's natural cellular processes of communication. Trehalose helps protect against cell stress and improves neurological functions.

Q: Does Trehalose help in cellular communication like glycoproteins?
A:
i: Trehalose helps in the proper folding of proteins and it is the improper folding of proteins that is the cause for neurodegenerative challenges.
ii. Trehalose is used in the building blocks of glycolipids which are the communication devices inside the cell.
iii. Glycoprotein receptor sites are rooted in the cell membrane. Because Trehalose strengthens the cell membrane, it is believed these communication devices are more stable and erect.

Q: **I am diabetic. Should I use Trehalose as a sweetener?**

A: Trehalose has a very low insulin response and provides sustained energy. Most diabetics benefit by replacing their regular table sugar with Trehalose. Consult your physician.

Q: **I understand that regular sugar feeds cancer.**
Does Trehalose feed cancer?

A: Trehalose is stable in high acid conditions (low pH levels) and does not feed cancer like regular table sugar. Consult your physician. See Smart Sugars Lessons: http://forum.endowmentmed.org/index.php

Q: **How is Trehalose unique?**

A: Trehalose is a multi-functional non-reducing disaccharide consisting of two glucose molecules bonded by an α,α - 1, 1 glycosidic link and is non-hygroscopic (does not attract moisture), which results in a free-flowing dry crystal stable to 94% humidity. Trehalose is Low Cariogenicity and has been shown to have substantially reduced cariogenic potential compared with sucrose and can therefore be used in the formulation of 'kind to teeth' and 'toothfriendly' products but without the laxative effects of other low-cariogenic bulk sweeteners.

Q: **How does Trehalose compare to regular sugar?**

A: Trehalose is more expensive; however, health benefits greatly increase it value. Trehalose has known protein and cell membrane stabilizing capabilities and may preserve and protect multiple normal biological systems by protecting the cell proteins and assisting with the production of protein cluster aggregates. Trehalose is 45% as sweet as table sugar The book, **Change Your Sugar, Change Your Life** references 145 health challenges caused or compounded by regular sugar and 65 health benefits of Trehalose. Request a **FREE Download of the book at** http://DiabeticHope.com. A hard copy is available on Amazon.

Q: **What do you mean by saying, "Trehalose is a flavor enhancer?"**

A: MSG is the harmful flavor enhancer used in many foods. Trehalose can be used in small amounts to enhance the flavor of foods. Somehow, it also helps lower harsh bitter flavors.

✳ Read science papers on the educational website http://endowmentmed.org

The profits from the sale of Trehalose go toward additional research and education through The Endowment for Medical Research, Inc a 501(c)(3) non-profit faith based research and educational public charity.

One Smart Sugar

T R E H A L O S E

The sugar everyone would use if they only knew...™
LEAVES A FRESH CLEAN TASTE IN YOUR MOUTH ...

Ingredients: 100% Trehalose Food Grade - GM free   Net Wt. **5 lbs** (2.268 kg)
Contains no other substances and no equipment was used that previously processed or bagged wheat, gluten, soybeans, dairy, egg, fish/shellfish, peanuts or any tree nut.

**Packaged for: The Endowment for Medical Research, Inc.
P. O. Box 73089 Houston, Texas 77273 • 281-587-2020**

Trehalose is a multi-functional naturally occurring sugar about half as sweet as sucrose and has a clean profile with no after-taste. Trehalose is a white crystalline dihydrate powder produced from tapioco or other starch. It is a non-reducing disaccharide consisting of 2 glucose molecules bonded by an α,α - 1, 1 glycosidic link and stable at low pH (stable in high acid) conditions and is non-hygroscopic (does not attract moisture), which resulting in a free-flowing dry crystal stable to 94% humidity. It is made by a patented enzymatic process.

Trehalose is Low Cariogenicity and has been shown to have substantially reduced cariogenic potential compared with sucrose and can therefore be used in the formulation of 'kind to teeth' and 'toothfriendly' products but without the laxative effects of other low-cariogenic bulk sweeteners.

Trehalose has known protein and cell membrane stabilizing capabilities and may preserve and protect multiple normal biological systems by protecting the cell proteins and assisting with the production of protein cluster aggregates. Trehalose may maintain and help the body's natural cellular processes of protein turnover and reduce neurological cell stress. Trehalose has a very low insulin response and provides sustained energy.✳

Trehalose also enhances the flavor of foods and is determined to be generally recognized as safe (GRAS) for use in foods in general in accordance with the current good manufacturing practices. Trehalose is approved as a food in countries world wide. Many people recommend six tablespoons per day.

✳ Learn more at http://endowmentmed.org

Nutrition Facts: Serving Size 1 Tablespoon 9g (9,258mg)(0.327oz) Servings Per Container 85	
Amount Per Serving Calories 33 (3.6 calories per g)	
	% Daily Value*
Total Fat 0g	0%
Potassium 0g	0%
Sodium 0mg	0%
Total Carbohydrates 8.33g	2.4%
Sugars 9g	
Protein 0g	0%

*Percentage Daily Values are based on a 2000 calorie diet. Your daily value may be higher or lower depending on your calorie needs. Caution: Any amount over 34 grams per day has not yet been determined safe by the FDA or USDA. Further testing is ongoing to discover the safe upper limits for human consumption, sustained energy, and other possible health benefits.

These statements have not been evaluated by the Food and Drug Administration. This product is not promoted to diagnose, treat, cure, or prevent any disease.

 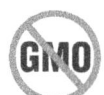

**The profit from this sale goes to
The Endowment for Medical Research, Inc.
a 501(c)(3) non-profit public charity**

Introducing a New Culinary Science

Our **Sugar Science Forum** has generated tens of thousands of hit as individuals have probed for uses of Trehalose.

Pat Champion posted:
It has been a while since I have posted anything but I just had to let everyone know that I am trying new recipes so I can use less sugar and in its place I am using Trehalose. We absolutely loved these cookies: TreHealthy Oatmeal Cookies

1½ cup whole wheat flour
3/4 teaspoon baking powder
1 teaspoon soda
2 cups oats
2 teaspoons cinnamon
1 1/2 cups Trehalose
1 teaspoon salt
3/4 cup ground flaxseed meal
Mix all dry ingredients together

3 egg whites
1 teaspoon vanilla
1 tablespoon cider vinegar
Beat together into dry ingredients until blended;
add 1-5 oz pack dried cherries
4 oz Ghirardelli 60% chocolate chips
3/4 cups nuts
Mix well and drop by teaspoons onto olive oiled cookie sheet. Bake at 375 degrees about 8 minutes.

Join the Champion family in our Heart TreHealthy Oatmeal Cookies!! They taste great!

Trehalose is a healthful replacement for MSG, simply makes things taste better, and helps make things last longer.

Trehalose overall acceptance increases and now meat processors include Trehalose in the curing process.

Bass Pro shops have started marketing the key ingredient for processing wild game. That secret ingredient is Trehalose. It improves the taste and appearance of homemade sausage, even eliminate that "freezer flavor" after freezing. Trehalose is a natural sweetener and anti-oxidant. It takes the "wild" out of game, "fishy" out of fish and "fowl" out of turkey sausage. Use 6 oz for 25 pounds of meat or 1½ teaspoons per pound. Use with fresh or cured sausages. Add with seasoning and water or directly blend with the meat.

A small amount of trehalose in foods has a very protective function where it has more benefits than just enhancing taste, being tooth friendly, and serving as a very healthful sugar. Trehalose seems to be the solution for refrigerated foods that form pools of water. Certain foods form pools of water when they are cooled, frozen, or defrosted.

Trehalose improves the flavor of appetizers, soups, sauces, meats, poultry, fish, vegetables, charcuterie, entrees, breads, pastries, desserts and hot and cold drinks.

Apply 1½ teaspoons of trehalose per pound of hamburger meat. Simple blend the trehalose directly into the meat. This will help if you are going to eat the hamburger today or plan to freeze patties for later. Use the trehalose before freezing the beef to eliminate the freezer flavor. This makes a great hamburger even better.

CONFECTIONARY
TREHALOSE

<u>Confectionary Trehalose is available nowhere else.</u>

Confectionary Trehalose improves the flavor of all fruit and desserts and makes them last longer. Makes for Great Nutrition Fun and leaves a good taste in your mouth.

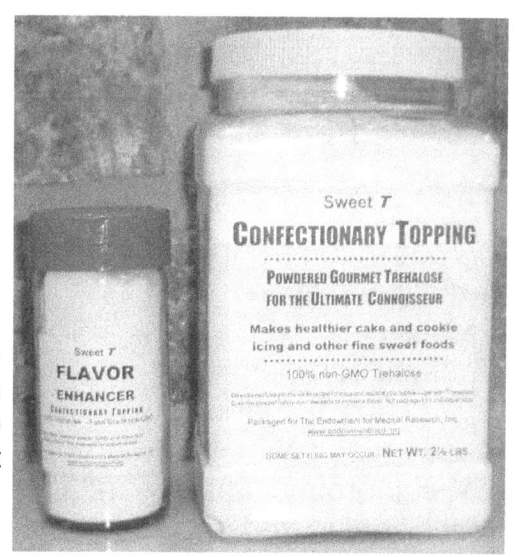

Never before has such a delicious healthful Confectionary sugar been available to the public. Never before has a Confectionary sugar been available that is so safe for children and adults. Imagine cake icing so wonderful, yet **knowing it is good for your health.** Test Confectionary Trehalose to make most fruit last a week longer.

Do the taste test for yourself. Take a small amount (1/4 teaspoon) of Confectionary Trehalose and taste the clean elongated sweetness. Cleanse you mouth with clean water and then do the same with regular store bought confectionary sugar. You will be shocked at the bitter aftertaste of regular confectionary sugar that is used for making virtually all cake icing.

Sweet T Confectionary Topping is 100% Pure Trehalose, a naturally occurring sugar about 45% as sweet as sucrose with a clean profile (no after-taste) and cleaner longer lasting sweetness than sucrose or any other confectionary sugar. **Sweet T Confectionary Topping** is a white crystalline dihydrate powder produced from tapioca or other non-GM starch. It is a non-reducing disaccharide consisting of two glucose molecules bonded by an α,α - 1, 1 glycosidic link which is stable at low pH conditions and is non-hygroscopic, which results in a free-flowing dry crystal that is stable to 94% humidity. It is made by a patented enzymatic process. **Sweet T Confectionary Topping** is Low Cariogenicity and has been shown to have substantially reduced cariogenic potential compared with sucrose and can therefore be used in the formulation of 'kind to teeth' and 'tooth friendly' products but without the laxative effects of other low-cariogenic sweeteners. **Sweet T Confectionary Topping** has known protein and cell membrane stabilizing capabilities and may preserve and protect multiple normal biological systems by protecting the cell proteins and interfering with the natural cellular processes of protein turnover and reduce neurological cell stress.

Introducing

SWEETER TREHALOSE

S W E E T E R than table sugar

The sugar everyone would use if they only knew...™

Now, you can enjoy the benefits of Trehalose with greater sweetness.
Use less Trehalose to SWEETEN your food and drink.

2 pound canister	$ 19.97
6 pound canister	$ 59.97
10 oz. Trial size	$ 7.77

Organic Stevia Rebaudiana (*Bertoni*) leaf powder is used to enhance the sweetness of Sweeter Trehalose. Stevia Rebaudiana adds no calories and is reported to not cause blood sugar spikes. Stevoa Rebaudiana (*Bertoni*) is prized Stevia that contains a high level of steviol glycosides with antioxidant, antimicrobial, and antifungal properties stable in high temperatures. You can cook with Sweeter Trehalose but over 250 degrees F may result in a slagging affect that produces a "grainy" texture in some baked foods. Enjoy cooking with Sweeter Trehalose to prepare the healthiest of dishes. Stevoa Rebaudiana (*Bertoni*) analysis has shown that it contains folic acid, vitamin C and all of the indispensable amino acids with the exception of tryptophan. Quality control with the very best makes for Sweeter Trehalose.

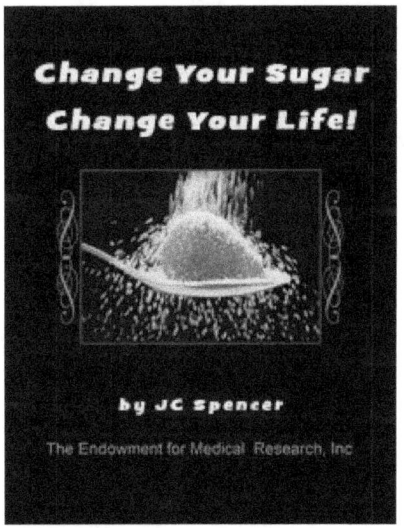

Change Your Sugar, Change Your LIFE
is an easy to read book for the student while packed with new information for
the seasoned medical professional,
research scientist, and learned professor.

Available on Amazon or downloadable at
http://DiabeticHope.com

What is the pH Fusion Tea Pilot Survey Matched Funding?

pH Fusion Tea

The FUSION SOLUTION

Designed to improve health and...

- inhibit fat cell enlargement
- inhibit inflammatory conditions
- strengthen cell membrane
- nourish the mitochondria
- eliminate acid reflux
- offset acid overload
- anti-depressant benefits
- metabolic syndrome
- protect cell proteins
- inhibit beta-amyloid 40 & 42
- absorb needed ionic multi-trace minerals
- inhibit progression of Type 2 Diabetes
- improve human cellular pH balance
- have superior nutrient absorption
- nourish neurological processes
- delay neurological malfunction
- delay onset of muscular dystrophy, MS, Parkinson's, Alzheimer's, ALS and Huntington's.

- brain function
- weight loss
- sustain energy
- lower triglycerides
- balance electrolytes
- heart burn
- stress tolerance
- body hydration
- help protein folding
- diabetes 1 & 2

These statements have not been evaluated by the Food and Drug Administration. This product is not promoted to diagnose, treat, cure, or prevent any disease.

Multiple University Research Studies in various countries verify that the functional components used in the design of pH Fusion Tea are known to have significant health benefits. Evidence of synergy or counter-synergy effect has not been determined. The health benefits may be unique to the individual and others may or may not receive similar benefits. In our research, we continue to have slow-responders, hyper-responders and non-responders. Our objective is to determine ways and means to continue to have improved results and to provide safety that is free from any drug side effects.

What are the Health Benefits of **pH Fusion Tea**?

By JC Spencer

The short answer is: "*We don't know.*" But, we are asking physicians, researcher, and the general public to participate in our pH Fusion Tea Nutritional Pilot Survey to discover if there are synergistic benefits superior to the studies already conducted on the individual functional ingredients.

The **pH Fusion Tea** components include the sugar trehalose, a natural buffer and carrier designed to help transport the bio-available ionic multi-trace minerals in a fulvic phytochemical compound through the cell membrane to stoke the mitochondria .

Separately, the components are noted for remarkable health benefits. Research papers are published and many posted on our website on the functional sugar trehalose at http://endowmentmed.org.

pH Fusion Tea as recommended is designed to help the cells have a higher pH, to receive better absorption of nutrients, and to better hydrate the human body.

Some trace minerals play significant roles in the reproduction and transcription of your DNA. Some of these are known as monoatomic or single atom minerals in the platinum mineral family (Iridium, Ruthenium, Rhodium, Palladium, Osmium, and Platinum). These and a few other monoatomic trace elements outside the Platinum family include silver and chromium. Some of these have a positive effect on plant cells, animals cells, and human cells. Other trace minerals that are not of the Platinum family nor are they monpatomic but still play roles in the DNA include phosphorus which, with a sugar, makes the back bone structure of the DNA's double helix. As research continues into the function of DNA, RNA, and mitochondria, we will learn more about the role of the trace minerals. Expect scientists to soon discover remarkable functions of mineral ions that have major health benefits for the human body.

The trace minerals in pH Fusion Tea include: antimony, barium, beryllium, bismuth, boron, bromine, calcium, carbon, cerium, cesium, chloride, chromium, cobalt, copper, dysprosium, erbium, europium, fluorine, gadolinium, gallium, germanium, gold, hafnium, holmium, indium, iodine, iridium, iron, lanthanum, lithium, lutetium, magnesium, manganese, molybdenum, neodymium, niacin, nickel, niobium, osmium, palladium, phosphorous, platinum, potassium, praseodymium, rhenium, rhodium, rubidium, ruthenium, samarium, scandium, selenium, silicon, silver, sodium, strontium, sulfur, tantalum, tellurium, terbium, thallium, thorium, thulium, tin, titanium, tungsten, vanadium, ytterbium, zinc, zirconium in a fulvic acid phytochemical compound.

The reasoning and potential for using pH Fusion Tea

pH Fusion Tea as recommended is designed to help the cells have a higher pH, to receive better absorption of nutrients, and to better hydrate the human body.

Trace Minerals and Your DNA

Some trace minerals play significant roles in the reproduction and transcription of your DNA. Some of these are known as monoatomic or single atom minerals in the platinum mineral family (Iridium, Ruthenium, Rhodium, Palladium, Osmium, and Platinum). These and a few other monoatomic trace elements outside the Platinum family include silver and chromium. Some of these have a positive effect on plant cells, animals cells, and human cells. Other trace minerals that are not of the Platinum family nor are they monpatomic but still play roles in the DNA include phosphorus which, with a sugar, makes the back bone structure of the DNA's double helix. As research continues into the function of DNA, RNA, and mitochondria, we will learn more about the role of the trace minerals. Expect scientists to soon discover remarkable functions of mineral ions that have major health benefits for the human body.

Mark Twain said, "*The difference between the right word and the almost-right word is the difference between the lightning and the lightning-bug.*"

Are trace minerals considered by most no more important than a lightning-bug? After reading The Trehalose Handbook Vol 1 & 2, you may agree with me, trace minerals are the lightning!

The trace minerals in pH Fusion Tea are the lightning!
antimony, barium, beryllium, bismuth, boron, bromine, calcium, carbon, cerium, cesium, chloride, chromium, cobalt, copper, dysprosium, erbium, europium, fluorine, gadolinium, gallium, germanium, gold, hafnium, holmium, indium, iodine, iridium, iron, lanthanum, lithium, lutetium, magnesium, manganese, molybdenum, neodymium, niacin, nickel, niobium, osmium, palladium, phosphorous, platinum, potassium, praseodymium, rhenium, rhodium, rubidium, ruthenium, samarium, scandium, selenium, silicon, silver, sodium, strontium, sulfur, tantalum, tellurium, terbium, thallium, thorium, thulium, tin, titanium, tungsten, vanadium, ytterbium, zinc, zirconium in a fulvic acid phytochemical compound.

For a limited time, you are welcome to download *The Trehalose Handbook Vol 1 and Vol 2* from our Download Store at no charge. Softbound editions are $29.95 each or both for $39.95.
http://endowmentmed.org/content/view/957/ The importance of the design of **pH Fusion Tea** is explained.

http://endowmentmed.org

Instructions for the pH Fusion Tea Nutritional Pilot Survey

Thank you for requesting information about participation in the self funding pH Fusion Tea Nutritional Pilot Survey.

Agreement:
Reviewing and submitting the **Baseline Health Evaluation Forms** acknowledges agreement for participating in the **pH Fusion Tea Pilot Survey** and a commitment to complete an Evaluation Form every 30 days during the Six Month Period.

Download the General Health Evaluation Form:
http://endowmentmed.org/pdf/GHE_FORM_pH_Fusion_Tea.pdf

Directions:
The pH Fusion Tea is a dry powder and must NOT be eaten dry or mixed with anything except clean water. Never mix with juices. It is best to use 2 Tablespoons per day, but at lease one heaping Tablespoon per day is needed for the study.

Mix 1 Tablespoon pH **Fusion Tea**™ in 4 to 8 ounces of clean filtered hot or cold water. [Use 1 heaping Tablespoon for faster response with more or less water to suit taste.] Take between meals, first morning drink and/or last evening drink, or as directed by physician. The taste is slightly sweet with a pleasant soothing swallow. (Beneficial to hold in mouth for a minute before swallowing.) You may add another teaspoon of trehalose for a sweeter taste. Do not take more than ten (10) Tablespoons of pH **Fusion Tea**™ **within a 24 hour period**, four (4) Tablespoons if you are over 60 years of age. Do not use the maximum amounts for more than two (2) weeks. It is recommended that your pH be monitored. You can monitor your saliva pH with a pH meter or pH strips. Saliva should test close to 7 pH.

More Information:
The pH factor of the liquid pH **Fusion Tea**™ is 9.5 but may vary slightly due to the pH factor of the water used.

pH Fusion Tea

with bio-available ionic multi-trace minerals in a dry phytochemical fulvic acid compound electrostatically blended in sodium

· ·

Designed to help human cells achieve a moderately higher pH; **have superior nutrient absorption; provide better body hydration; absorb needed ionic multi-trace minerals.**

· ·

Packaged for The Endowment for Medical Research Inc
P. O. Box 73089 - Houston, Texas 77273 (281) 587-2020 - FAX (281) 397-6789
a 501(c)(3) non-profit faith based scientific research, educational, Public Charity.
Non-Profit Tax ID # 54-2073489   DUNS # 140133815
Profits used for Medical Research, Educational Research, and Education
http://endowmentmed.org

pH *Fusion Tea*™ is a proprietary nutritional buffer designed to help raise and modulate the human cellular pH level, to lower acid level, and reduce cell stress. pH *Fusion Tea*™ is designed to offset acid overload without interrupting good digestion. The buffer formulation is designed to fortify the cell membrane and to equip the cell for superior nutrient absorption.

pH *Fusion Tea*™ is a specific blend of trehalose, sodium bicarbonate, and ionic micro-nutrient multi-trace minerals. Trehalose is a multi-functional naturally occurring sugar about 45% as sweet as sucrose and has a clean profile. Trehalose is a white crystalline dihydrate powder produced from tapioca / starch. It is a non-reducing disaccharide consisting of two glucose molecules bonded by an α,α - 1, 1 glycosidic link which is **stable at low pH (high acid) conditions** and is non-hygroscopic (moisture attraction), which results in a free-flowing dry crystal that is stable to 94% humidity. Trehalose has known protein and cell membrane stabilizing capabilities designed to preserve and protect multiple normal biological systems by protecting the cell proteins and interfering with the natural cellular processes of protein turnover and reduce neurological cell stress. Trehalose has a very low insulin response and provides sustained energy.

The Buffer, sodium bicarbonate, is a naturally occurring substance that is found in all living things, where it helps modulate (regulate) their pH balance. The Buffer is made from soda ash, which is mined in the form of an ore called trona. The soda ash is then dissolved into a solution through which carbon dioxide is bubbled and sodium bicarbonate precipitates out, forming the "Pure, Safe and Natural" Buffer.

Warnings: Do not use if you are on a sodium restricted diet unless directed by a doctor. Ask a doctor or a pharmacist before use if you are taking a prescription drug. pH *Fusion Tea*™ acts as an antacid and certain prescription drugs may interact with it. Do not administer to children under age 5. STOMACH WARNING: TO AVOID SERIOUS INJURY, DO NOT TAKE UNTIL POWDER IS COMPLETELY DISSOLVED in water. IT IS VERY IMPORTANT NOT TO TAKE THIS PRODUCT DRY OR WHEN OVERLY FULL FROM FOOD OR DRINK. Consult a doctor if severe stomach pain occurs after taking this product. Stop use and ask a doctor should symptoms last more than 2 weeks. Mix only with clean filtered water. DO NOT add a different sweetener, juice, or other ingredients as that may upset the pH balance.

pH *Fusion Tea*™ contains **NO** Baking Powder which is a mixture of baking soda and various acidic ingredients which makes a carbon dioxide producing reaction.

Directions: Mix 2 ½ tsp pH *Fusion Tea*™ in 4 to 5 ounces of clean filtered hot or cold water. [Use 4 teaspoons for faster response with more water to suit taste.] Take between meals, first morning drink & last evening drink, or as directed by physician. The taste is slightly sweet with a pleasant soothing swallow. (Beneficial to hold in mouth for a minute before swallowing.) You may add another teaspoon of trehalose for a sweeter taste. Do not take more than twenty eight (28) teaspoons of pH *Fusion Tea*™ within a 24 hour period, twelve (12) teaspoons if you are over 60 years of age. Do not use the maximum amounts for more than two (2) weeks. It is recommended that your pH be monitored. You can monitor your saliva pH with a pH meter or pH strips. Saliva should test close to 7 pH.

Other Information: Each teaspoon contains 154 mg sodium. pH *Fusion Tea*™ is designed to help resist radical changes in pH balance - this is called buffering. When pH *Fusion Tea*™ comes in contact with either an acidic or an alkaline substance, it's natural effect is to modulate (neutralize) extreme pH level. Two and ½ tea-spoons of pH *Fusion Tea*™ in 4 to 6 oz of clean filtered hot or cold water has a factor of over 9 pH. The pH factor of the liquid pH *Fusion Tea*™ may vary slightly due to the pH factor of the water used.

Ingredients: Trehalose (Food Grade), sodium bicarbonate, and ionic multi-trace minerals in a phytochemical fulvic acid compound.

These statements have not been evaluated by the Food and Drug Administration. This product is not intended to diagnose, treat, cure, or prevents any disease.

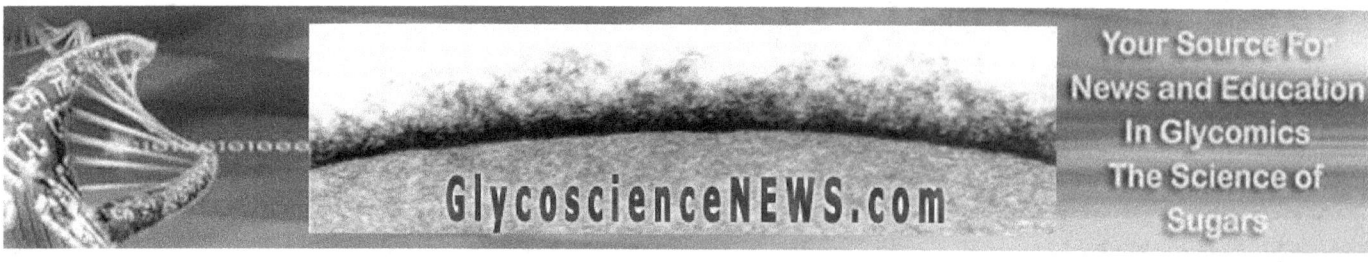

Why is pH Fusion Tea So Unbelievably Functional?

Research scientists learn more about the mystery of the possible fusion solution: pH, fusion, ion gates, glucose/sodium transport, Trehalose and how neurological benefits are achieved to improve mental clarity, Alzheimer's, Parkinson's, MS and ALS

by JC Spencer

Before we answer the question: *"Why is pH Fusion Tea So Unbelievably Functional?"*, we need to answer: *"What is pH Fusion Tea?"*

> pH Fusion Tea is a blend of propriety functional food ingredients designed to support the mitochondria. The ingredients include the sugar Trehalose, sodium and ~80 charged trace minerals electrostatically blended. The design is to first increase the pH environment outside the cell so as to trigger a pH increase inside the cell. Research has taught us that a slight increase in pH can open ion gates in the cell wall.

pH is NOT a Substance

pH is the measuring scale for how acidic or alkaline a substance is with a range of 0 to 14 with 7 as the pH neutral. The strong hydrochloric acid (muriatic acid) is 1. The strong alkaline sodium hydroxide (caustic soda (lye), is 14.

Slight Increase in pH is Important

As an electrolyte, pH Fusion Tea is designed to pass through the plasma membrane with one dietary inorganic macronutrient mineral and ~80 bio-available organic micronutrient trace minerals electrostatically blended. In fact, to increase the pH is to help open the ion gates so that the fuel can enter the cell.

Trehalose, a two molecule sugar, is

a multi-functional disaccharide consisting of two glucose molecules with a unique stabilizing bond. Trehalose strengthens the cell membrane. Unlike other sugars, it can withstand a strong acid environment and research shows that Trehalose can block electron beam radiation.

Health benefits are widely reported for Trehalose, especially from those with neurological challenges including problems with mental clarity, Parkinson's, Huntington's, MS and ALS. Trehalose is the base ingredient of pH Fusion Tea. We are receiving "unbelievable" functional reports on this "Tea" designed to support and stoke the mitochondria and strengthen the human cell membrane.

When I formulated pH Fusion Tea with Trehalose, I perceived a part of the potential efficacy it could have in the human body. It was highly significant to understanding that Trehalose is stable in an acid environment while also working well in an alkaline environment.

Trehalose Works Well with Alkaline-Earth Metal Ions

A team of researchers in Okayama, Japan investigated and published a paper entitled: *"Interaction between Trehalose and alkaline-earth metal ions."* The nuclear relaxation times of carbon atoms of Trehalose were shortened by addition of [certain] alkaline-earth chloride salts. Other research indicates that Trehalose forms metal-complexes with the alkaline-earth metal[s].

In Parts Two through Four, we will discuss:
- Trace Minerals and Your DNA ▪ Ion Gates ▪ ATP is
- Mitochondria Power Generators ▪ Fusion results
- Designed to Transport Trace Minerals to the Cell
- Designed to Open Ion Gates in the Cell Wall
- The Glucose/Sodium Transport System and HOW IT WORKS
- Explaining Ion Gates and ATP
- pH Fusion Tea is Designed to Support Red Blood Cells
- Vital Importance of Trace Minerals
- We invite others to research with us.

Sources and References

This lesson is a summary of the complex working of the Glucose/Sodium Transport System discussed in Chapter 6 of The Trehalose Handbook Vol. One; and, Chapter 10 of The Trehalose Handbook Vol. Two entitled
"A Quick Study of the Importance of Trace Minerals in the Human Body".
Change your Sugar - Change Your Life www.DiabeticHope.com
www.PilotStudies.net
www.GlycoscienceNEWS.com www.Glycosciencewhitepaper.com
SMART SUGARS www.OneSmartSugar.com/video.html
Expand Your Mind - Improve Your Brain
http://www.endowmentmed.org/ExpandYourMind/MindEbook3.html
Glycoscience Lesson #33 Part One of Four
http://www.GlycoscienceNEWS.com/pdf/Lesson33PartOneOfFour.pdf
http://EzineArticles.com/?expert=JC_Spencer
© The Endowment for Medical Research www.endowmentmed.org

GlycoscienceNEWS.com

Your Source For News and Education In Glycomics The Science of Sugars

Why is pH Fusion Tea So Unbelievably Functional?

Research scientists learn more about the mystery of the possible fusion solution: pH, fusion, ion gates, glucose/sodium transport, Trehalose and how neurological benefits are achieved to improve mental celerity, Alzheimer's, Parkinson's, MS and ALS

by JC Spencer

Trace Minerals and Your DNA

Some trace minerals play significant roles in the DNA. Some of these are known as monoatomic or single atom minerals in the platinum mineral family (Iridium, Ruthenium, Rhodium, Palladium, Osmium, and Platinum). A few other monoatomic trace elements outside the Platinum family includes chromium and silver. Some of these have significant positive effect on human cells. Other trace minerals that are not monpatomic still play roles in the DNA. Phosphorus binds with a sugar to make the back bone structure of the DNA's double helix. As research continues into the function of DNA, RNA, and the mitochondria, we will learn more about the role of the trace minerals. Expect scientists to soon discover remarkable functions of mineral ions that will have major health benefits for the human body.

Ion Gates are water-filled ion pores in the cell wall. These portals can transport hydrophilic molecules through cell walls.

ATP is adenosine triphosphate, the final fuel to metabolize energy in the cell. The mitochondria generates energy in an aerobic cycle utilizing oxygen. The cell breaks down glucose and produces waste as carbon dioxide and water. Each molecule of glucose makes ~36 molecules of ATP. A shortage of oxygen can restrict ATP production to two molecules. The "clean" quality and quantity of ATP regulates cellular signals that control the human body. Impure final fuel can produce "dirty" electricity that results in free radical damage to cells. Trehalose provides sustained glucose energy to make ATP. Ionic micro trace minerals in pH Fusion Tea is designed to stoke the mitochondria.

Mitochondria Power Generators

These tiny generator powerhouses within the cell produce electricity that powers the mental and motor functions of the body. The electron microscope reveals that some cells contain many, even thousands of various shaps and sizes of mitochondria. Scientists do not yet understand how these generators work but their design is believed to be beyond the technology and sophistication of any power source man has developed.

Designed to Transport Trace Minerals Into the Cell

Two forms of transports pass nutrients through the plasma membrane into the cell. Each transport system seeks the path of least resistance. When glucose moves across the cell membrane (through the cell wall), it travels from the higher concentrated area outside the cell to the lower concentrated area inside the cell. This **Passive transport** process is osmosis by diffusion that requires no energy. The **Active transport** process requires energy to reverse the pathway so glucose is transported from the lower to higher concentrated area. The design of pH Fusion Tea is to facilitate Active Transport.

In Parts Three and Four, we will discuss:
- Fusion results ■ Designed to Open Ion Gates in the Cell Wall
- The Glucose/Sodium Transport System and HOW IT WORKS
- Explaining Ion Gates and ATP
- pH Fusion Tea is Designed to Support Red Blood Cells
- Vital Importance off Trace Minerals
- We invite others to research with us.
- Sources and References

Sources and References

This lesson is a summary of the complex working of the Glucose/Sodium Transport System discussed in Chapter 6 of The Trehalose Handbook Vol. One and Chapter 10 of The Trehalose Handbook Vol. Two entitled "A Quick Study of the Importance of Trace Minerals in the Human Body".

Change your Sugar - Change Your Life www.DiabeticHope.com www.PilotStudies.net

www.GlycoscienceNEWS.com
www.Glycosciencewhitepaper.com

SMART SUGARS   www.OneSmartSugar.com/video.html

Expand Your Mind - Improve Your Brain
http://www.endowmentmed.org/ExpandYourMind/MindEbook3.html

Glycoscience Lesson #33 Part Two of Four
http://www.GlycoscienceNEWS.com/pdf/Lesson33PartTwoOfFour.pdf

http://EzineArticles.com/?expert=JC_Spencer

GlycoscienceNEWS.com

Your Source For
News and Education
In Glycomics
The Science of
Sugars

Why is pH Fusion Tea So Unbelievably Functional?

Research scientists learn more about the mystery of the possible fusion solution:
pH, fusion, ion gates, glucose/sodium transport, Trehalose and how neurological
benefits are achieved to improve mental celerity, Alzheimer's, Parkinson's, MS and ALS

by JC Spencer

Glycoscience Lesson #33
Part Three of Four

Fusion results

from the process of combining multiple distinct entities into a new whole. Fusion results in a new function beyond the individual components.

How to Open Ion Gates in the Cell Wall

The ion gates are opened and closed by signals according to the needs of the cell and the environment around the cell. A slight increase in the pH environment around the cell can open ion gates.

Transmembrane proteins create water-filled ion pores which can transport hydrophilic molecules. Glycolipids (inside the cell) and glycoproteins (on the cell surface) provide the communication. Specific Smart Sugars are the building blocks for the glycolipids and glycoproteins with Trehalose, when present, assisting in the proper folding of the proteins. Improper folding of the proteins is the cause for all neurodegenerative challenges.

The Glucose/Sodium transport system and HOW IT WORKS

The pH Fusion Tea design is to enable molecules to pass through the membrane by a conformational change in the shape of the transmembrane protein when it binds with the molecule to be transported.

Glucose and sodium couple to form a co-transport system that uses the positively charged sodium ions which are attracted to the negative area to increase the higher concentration on the outside of the cell.

Explaining Ion Gates and ATP

Voltage gated channels allow sodium into the cell and similar channels let potassium out of the cell. Transporters use ATP energy to move ions and small molecules through the membrane. Flow of current through a single ion gate has been measured with the patch clamp technique at ~7,000 sodium ions transported within ~1 millisecond that the gate is open.

Neurons and muscle cells have a negative membrane potential. The inside of the cell is more negative than the outside with the propensity to push sodium outside.

Sodium ions build an electrostatic charge on the cell membrane. ATP pumps ions uphill against their electro-chemical gradients through the membrane by a special protein enzyme known as sodium potassium ATPase that serves as a pumping mechanism. This process occurs within the cell for optimal distribution of cellular chemicals.

Action potential conducts an electrical impulse as the positive charge flows toward negative charge. As the membrane is made more permeable to sodium, it rushes INTO the cell like a speeding bullet.

Negatively charged proteins are manufactured inside the cell. Proteins within the cell membrane transport glucose. Due to the electrochemical gradient, sodium enters a binding site specific for it on the protein, and when this is accomplished, the protein changes its shape (allosteric reaction), so that sodium can bind and be transported into the cell. This co-transport of multiple substances is transported into the cell together. To take in the proper amount of sodium, we increase the concentration gradient outside of the cell and therefore increase sodium's ability to bind to transport proteins.

In Part Four, we will discuss:
- pH Fusion Tea is Designed to Support Red Blood Cells
- Vital Importance of Trace Minerals
- We invite others to research with us.
- Sources and References

Sources and References

This lesson is a summary of the complex working of the Glucose/Sodium Transport System discussed in Chapter 6 of The Trehalose Handbook Vol. One and Chapter 10 of The Trehalose Handbook Vol. Two entitled "A Quick Study of the Importance of Trace Minerals in the Human Body".

Change your Sugar - Change Your Life www.DiabeticHope.com
www.PilotStudies.net

www.GlycoscienceNEWS.com www.Glycosciencewhitepaper.com
SMART SUGARS www.OneSmartSugar.com/video.html
Expand Your Mind - Improve Your Brain
http://www.endowmentmed.org/ExpandYourMind/MindEbook3.html
Glycoscience Lesson #33 Part Three of Four
http://www.GlycoscienceNEWS.com/pdf/Lesson33PartThreeOfFour.pdf
http://EzineArticles.com/?expert=JC_Spencer
© The Endowment for Medical Research www.endowmentmed.org

GlycoscienceNEWS.com

Your Source For
News and Education
In Glycomics
The Science of
Sugars

Why is pH Fusion Tea So Unbelievably Functional?

Research scientists learn more about the mystery of the possible fusion solution: pH, fusion, ion gates, glucose/sodium transport, Trehalose and how neurological benefits are achieved to improve mental celerity, Alzheimer's, Parkinson's, MS and ALS

by JC Spencer

Glycoscience Lesson #33
Part Four of Four

pH Fusion Tea is designed to support red blood cells:

Plasma membrane of human red blood cells contain transmembrane proteins that permit the diffusion of glucose from blood into the cell. While I believe that pH Fusion Tea facilitates diffusion of the microtrace minerals, this has not yet been proven to my satisfaction.

Vital Importance of Trace Minerals

Trace minerals are crucial for body functions in every aspect of life and maintenance and in the repair of tissues and bones. Scientists do not yet understand the function of all the trace minerals because some are used in extremely small amounts to do extremely important functions in their reacting with each other.

There is greater importance to the valence electrons, the electron affinity, the atomic number, the atomic weight, the molar volume, the stability of the isotopes, the ionization energies (the least required energy to release a single electron from the atom), electron configuration, the electronegativity, the ionic radius and other factors. Medical science understands very little about what all this means and how these influences impact the human cell.

Properly utilized, trace minerals may prove to be one of the most significant scientific discoveries of modern time. Balance is the key. Modulation and balance are attained by trace elements and proper nutrition.

Trace elements are nanoparticles or nanopowders. In **The Trehalose Handbook Volume Two**, I discuss the health benefits of ~80 trace minerals in pH Fusion Tea. Here we will "glance" at sodium which is not to be confessed with too much salt which is the source of compounding health problems. Sodium is an electrolyte and one of its functions is to pass through the cell membrane. The Structure Function of sodium plays a deciding role in cellular metabolism. Sodium, an inorganic nutrient, unlike other minerals, penetrates the cell membrane and modulates the pH which is vital to all metabolism. Other inorganic minerals do not easily absorb into the human cell. Sodium is an alkali metal, unique and vital. It has an atomic number 11, an atomic weight: 22.98976928, a positive charge +1. Sodium with potassium flows back and forth across cell membranes to maintain homeostasis in the cell. Salt and sodium are not the same thing. Table salt is 40 percent sodium and 60 percent chloride. Sodium bicarbonate contains no chloride. It is the chloride with the sodium that causes more problems. Sodium balance is brought by other minerals and tract minerals including potassium, magnesium, and calcium. The balance of sodium and water in the body can be disrupted if there is not enough water. Without sodium, nerves and muscles would cease to function, the absorption of major nutrients would be impaired, and the body would not be able to maintain adequate water and mineral balance.

We Invite Others to Research with us

Physicians, nurses, and researchers are welcomed to assist in evaluation of their patients with health challenges especially neurological, including MS, ALS, Alzheimer's, Parkinson's and Huntington's, as well as diabetes who participate in a pH Fusion Tea Pilot Survey.

If you think this is complex or perplexing, wait until we understand the ~800,000 glycans and glycoproteins on the surface of each cell and how we can further influence their communication ability.

No cure or treatment claims are intended or implied. Reporting and publishing of educational material does not provide legal or personal advice. Readers should be aware that any educational information may contain inherent or potential risks and there is no guarantee of any kind. Any past performance does not assure the same future results and some information may be hypothetical. We encourage general financial contributions to help us cover operational expenses and designated contributions for specific studies, pilot surveys, or medical research projects concerning various ongoing research and discoveries as will be outlined upon request.

Sources and References

This lesson is a summary of the complex working of the Glucose/Sodium Transport System discussed in Chapter 6 of The Trehalose Handbook Vol. One and Chapter 10 of The Trehalose Handbook Vol. Two titled "A Quick Study of the Importance of Trace Minerals in the Human Body".

Change your Sugar - Change your Life www.DiabeticHope.com
www.PilotStudies.net

www.GlycoscienceNEWS.com www.Glycosciencewhitepaper.com
SMART SUGARS www.OneSmartSugar.com/video.html

Expand Your Mind - Improve Your Brain
http://www.endowmentmed.org/ExpandYourMind/MindEbook3.html
Glycoscience Lesson #33 Part Four of Four
http://www.GlycoscienceNEWS.com/pdf/Lesson33FourOfFour.pdf
http://EzineArticles.com/?expert=JC_Spencer
© The Endowment for Medical Research www.endowmentmed.org

What is the
T/C+ Pilot Survey
Matched Funding?

T/C+

- lower high blood pressure
- serve as an anti-depressant
- aid stress tolerance
- provide cardiovascular support
- inhibit fat cell enlargement
- strengthen cell membrane
- nourish neurological processes
- delay neurological malfunction

- aid brain function
- lower LDL cholesterol
- lower triglycerides
- aid metabolic syndrome
- reduce inflammation
- help overcome diabetes 1 & 2
- inhibit progression of Type 2 Diabetes
- inhibit progression of beta-amyloid 40 and 42

- reduce cell stress
- sustain energy
- reduce arthritis
- stabilize proteins
- help protein folding

http://PilotStudies.net

We welcome individuals with the following health challenged into a T/C+ Six Month Pilot Survey **because research shows that** T/C+ **may provide a higher quality of life and delay the onset of and sometimes may reverse certain neurological processes which include:**

muscular dystrophy ✔ **MS** ✔ **Parkinson's** ✔ **Alzheimer's** ✔ **ALS** ✔ **stroke** ✔

spina bifida ✔ **sleep apnea** ✔ **shingles** ✔ **peripheral neuropathy** ✔

muscular dystrophy ✔ **migraines** ✔ **meningitis** ✔ **Lyme's** ✔ **fibromyalgia** ✔ **epilepsy**

✔ **ADD** ✔ **encephalitis** ✔ **Down's syndrome** ✔ **dementia** ✔ **AdHD** ✔

chronic fatigue ✔ **bipolar** ✔ **autism** ✔ **alcoholism** ✔ and **Huntington's** ✔.

Multiple University Research Studies in various countries verify the functional components used in the design of T/C+ are known to have significant health benefits. Evidence of neither synergy nor counter-synergy effect has been determined. Health benefits are unique to individuals and others may or may not receive similar benefits. In our research, we continue to have slow-responders, hyper-responders and non-responders.

http://PilotStudies.net

Our objective is to discover ways and means to continue to improve health and to provide solutions with a DO NO HARM Safety policy in a drug free environment.

What are the Health Benefits of T/C+?

The short answer is: *"We don't know."* But, we are asking physicians, researcher, and the general public to participate in a Nutritional Pilot Survey to discover if there are synergistic benefits superior to the astounding studies already conducted on the individual functional ingredients.

T/C+ has three basic components, the sugar trehalose, Ceylon cinnamon, and bio-available ionic multi-trace minerals in a fulvic phytochemical compound.

Separately, the components are noted for remarkable health benefits. Research papers are published and many posted on our website on the functional sugar trehalose at http://endowmentmed.org. Cinnamon benefits have been known for centuries and include lowering blood fat and blood sugar levels, helping arthritis sufferers and preventing diabetes. Studies also show cinnamon has health benefits with triglycerides, total cholesterol and the 'bad' LDL cholesterol in those with type II diabetes. It is an aphrodisiac and anti-fungal agent and calms the nerves. **T/C+** contains only Ceylon cinnamon. [*There are warnings against using too much Cassia cinnamon (the cinnamon sold in grocery stores) because of its coumarin content which is toxic to the liver and kidneys and may cause damage even in small amounts*.] Now, about ionic trace minerals. We have reports from outside the US that research supports and governments approve the use of ionic multi-trace minerals for the treatment of cancer and viruses. How effective it is? We do not know.

The USDA modified a paper on 05/07/2011 how cinnamon effects the signaling proteins (That would be glycoproteins.) to decrease the risk for insulin resistance, heart disease, and cancer especially dealing with leukemic cells. That Abstract is available under sources.

Submit your request for more information about participating in the Pilot Survey.
http://endowmentmed.org/PilotSurvey

Sources include: the USDA
http://ncbi.nlm.nih.gov/pubmed/14709014

http://ars.usda.gov/research/publications/publications.htm?seq_no_115=202479

http://thermo.com/eThermo/CMA/PDFs/Various/File_1818.pdf

http://endowmentmed.org

Individuals may apply for Matched Funding for a national 6 Month Pilot Survey for any health condition listed here plus cancer. Applications will be considered at http://PilotStudies.net. Doctors and other healthcare professionals may help monitor participants but this is not required for participation. Matched Funding participation in the Pilot Survey may be provided anywhere in the world except where taxed or prohibited by law.

Instructions for the T/C+ Nutritional Pilot Survey

For those interesting in the self funding T/C+ Nutritional Pilot Survey.

Qualifications, Rules, and Evaluations

The Honor System is used in this Study. Because of the **Matched Funding**, the cost for the six month Study is very low. Participants may submit General Health Evaluation Forms; however, we are especially looking for individuals with the health challenges outlined in our announcement.
Http://endowmentmed.org/odf/TC+WhatAreBenefits5911

The Endowment for Medical Research, Inc covers half the cost. Each two pound container of T/C+ is for one month.

Full six month supply with **Matched Funding** is $177.70 plus shipping.

Agreement:

Reviewing and submitting the **Baseline General Health Evaluation** Form acknowledges agreement for participating in the **T/C+** Pilot Survey.

Download the General Health Evaluation Form:
http://endowmentmed.org/pdf/GHE_FORM_TC+.pdf

Directions: This is the Pilot Survey designed for the participant to enjoy. Use enough T/C+ to flavor for best enjoyment. It is desirable to consume 2 Tablespoons per day; BUT, it is very important to eat at least 1 Tablespoon. So enjoy the amount that you believe is best for you. Even a smaller amount is much better than none. Enjoy T/C+ on toast and on your cereal. Here are great ways of enjoying T/C+: Enrich apple butter or apple sauce by stirring T/C+ into it. T/C+ improves oatmeal, cream of wheat, Malt-O-Meal, and other hot cereals. Sprinkle it on your ice cream or whipping cream. Sprinkle it on your pancakes and waffles. Sprinkle on your salad. Fruit pies baked with T/C+ instead of regular sugar makes for the best mouth watering home made pie you ever ate. Or, take any ready-made apple pie and sprinkle lots of T/C+ on top. Add to pears, rhubarb, puddings, and custards. Add to your hot chocolate or in your coffee. Be creative and share your recipes with us. [Warning: T/C+ does not mix well in liquids without additional stirring.]

Explaining T/C+

T/C+ has three basic components, the sugar trehalose, Ceylon cinnamon, and bio-available ionic multi-trace minerals in a fulvic phytochemical compound.

Separately, the components are noted for remarkable health benefits. Research papers are published and many posted on our website on the functional sugar trehalose at http://endowmentmed.org. Cinnamon benefits have been known for centuries and include lowering blood fat and sugar levels, helping arthritis sufferers and preventing diabetes. Studies also show cinnamon has health benefits with triglycerides, total cholesterol and the 'bad' LDL cholesterol in those with type II diabetes. It is an aphrodisiac and anti-fungal agent and calms the nerves. T/C+ contains only Ceylon cinnamon. [*There are warnings against using too much Cassia cinnamon (the cinnamon sold in grocery stores) because of its coumarin content which is toxic to the liver and kidneys and may cause damage even in small amounts.*] We have reports from outside the US that research supports and governments approve the use of ionic multi-trace minerals for the treatment of cancer and viruses. How effective it is? We do not know. This is the reason for the Pilot Survey prior to additional clinical trials. Your participation is appreciated and very important to ongoing education, improvement of healthcare, and the lowering of healthcare costs.

Individuals may apply for Matched Funding for a national 6 Month Pilot Survey for any health condition listed here plus cancer, Lyme's and depression. Applications will be considered at **http://PilotStudies.net**. Doctors and other healthcare professionals may help monitor participants but this is not required for participation. Matched Funding participation in the Pilot Survey may be provided anywhere in the world except where taxed or prohibited by law.

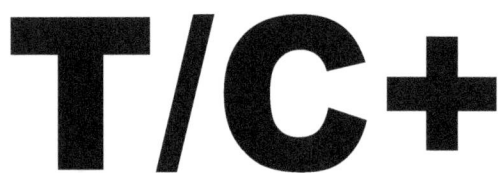

T/C+

· ·

**designed to enhance brain function and health
with fun filled flavor of cinnamon and
bio-available ionic multi-trace minerals**

· ·

Food Facts

Active ingredients

Trehalose, Ceylon cinnamon, and bio-available ionic multi-trace minerals in fulvic acid phytochemical compound including: antimony, barium, beryllium, bismuth, boron, bromine, calcium, carbon, cerium, cesium, chloride, chromium, cobalt, copper, dysprosium, erbium, europium, fluorine, gadolinium, gallium, germanium, gold, hafnium, holmium, indium, iodine, iridium, iron, lanthanum, lithium, lutetium, magnesium, manganese, molybdenum, neodymium, niacin, nickel, niobium, osmium, palladium, phosphorous, platinum, potassium, praseodymium, rhenium, rhodium, rubidium, ruthenium, samarium, scandium, selenium, silicon, silver, sodium, strontium, sulfur, tantalum, tellurium, terbium, thallium, thorium, thulium, tin, titanium, tungsten, vanadium, ytterbium, zinc, zirconium.

Uses

■ designed to temporarily protect cell membrane and nourish the body and improve cognitive function

Warning

■ Do not get in eyes

KEEP OUT OF REACH OF CHILDREN
If more than the recommended amount is swallowed at one time, get medical help or contact a Poison Control Center right away.

Nutrition Facts: Serving Size 1 Tablespoon (1oz) (14.7g)
Servings Per 2 lb Container 64

Amount Per Serving
Calories 42.65†(2.9 calories per g)

	% Daily Value*
Total Fat 0.04g	0.06%
Potassium 5.67mg	0.16%
Sodium 0mg	0%
Total Carbohydrates 7g	2%
Sugars 7.5g	
Protein 0.04g	0.08%
Dietary fiber 0.62g	2.48%
Calcium 13.92mg	1.39%
Iron 0.43mg	2.39%

*Percentage Daily Values are based on a 2000 calorie diet. Your daily value may be higher or lower depending on your calorie needs. †Trehalose is sustained energy and not immediately metabolized; therefore, less than 100% of the calories may be assimilated into the body as glucose resulting in a low insulin response. Caution: Any amount over (34g of trehalose per day has not yet been determined safe by the FDA or USDA. Further testing is ongoing to discover the safe upper limits for human consumption, sustained energy, and other possible health benefits.

T/C+ is a specific blend of trehalose, Ceylon cinnamon, and bio-available ionic micro-nutrient multi-trace minerals. Trehalose is a multi-functional naturally occurring sugar about 45% as sweet as sucrose and has a clean profile. Trehalose is a white crystalline dihydrate powder produced from tapioca / starch. It is a non-reducing disaccharide consisting of two glucose molecules bonded by an α,α - 1, 1 glycosidic link which is stable at low pH (high acid) conditions and is non-hygroscopic. Trehalose has known protein and cell membrane stabilizing capabilities designed to preserve and protect multiple normal biological systems by protecting the cell proteins and interfering with the natural cellular processes of protein turnover and reduce neurological cell stress. Trehalose has a low insulin response and provides sustained energy.

T/C+ contains the more expensive Ceylon cinnamon which is more preferred in Europe. Its flavor is quite distinct with a subtle complexity that you won't experience with the stronger, spicier cassia cinnamon. The light, intricate flavor of Ceylon cinnamon makes it the cinnamon of choice for many dishes such dishes as custards, ice cream, apples, pears, rhubarb, puddings, hot chocolate, and whipping cream. Cinnamon is a great source of manganese, fiber, iron, and calcium. Studies have shown that just ½ teaspoon of the cinnamon per day can lower LDL cholesterol. University studies indicate that cinnamon fights inflamation, relief from pain caused by infections, and may aid in protection from the E. coli bacteria.

Several studies suggest that **T/C+** may have a regulatory effect on blood sugar, making it especially beneficial for people with Type 2 diabetes. In a study at Copenhagen University, patients given half a teaspoon of cinnamon combined with one tablespoon of honey every morning before breakfast had significant relief in arthritis pain after one week and could walk without pain within one month.

T/C+ contains bio-available ionic multi-trace minerals in a fulvic acid phytochemical compound.

Warnings: Ask a doctor or a pharmacist before use if you are taking a prescription drug. Just because one person has beneficial health benefits does not mean that another will have benefit because each person has his or her unique body chemistry which may cause a different result. Do not administer to children under age 5. STOMACH WARNING: TO AVOID SERIOUS INJURY. Consult a doctor if severe stomach pain occurs after taking this product. Stop use and ask a doctor should symptoms last more than 2 weeks.

Directions: Sprinkle a minimum of 1 Tablespoon of **T/C+** on toast, muffin, cereal, salad, tea, coffee or other food per day. **T/C+** can be used to enhance many recipes while giving them a great quality beneficial to improved health.

Other Information: The Endowment for Medical Research, a non-profit faith-based scientific research and educational public charity, is conducting a self funding **T/C+** Six Month Pilot Survey to gather Evaluation Form Questionnaires from participants. Information and instructions for participation are available on website at http://endowmentmed.org. Ask how you or someone you love can participate and receive partial sponsorship.**100% Money Back Guarantee:** If for any reason a customer is not completely satisfied, her or she may call 281-587-2020, request an authorization number for a complete refund by returning the empty container any time within 180 days from purchase.

Packaged for The Endowment for Medical Research Inc
P. O. Box 73089 - Houston, Texas 77273 (281) 587-2020 - FAX (281) 397-6789
a 501(c)(3) non-profit faith based scientific research, educational, Public Charity.
Non-Profit Tax ID # 54-2073489 DUNS # 140133815
Profits used for Medical Research, Educational Research, and Education

http://endowmentmed.org

These statements have not been evaluated by the Food and Drug Administration. This product is not intended to diagnose, treat, cure, or prevents any disease.

Ingredients: Trehalose (Food Grade), Celyon cinnamon, and bio-available ionic multi-trace minerals in a phytochemical fulvic acid compound

New Findings: Dangers of the Wrong Cinnamon and Statin Drugs
Our T/C+ Pilot Surveys are more important than ever!

Glycoscience Lesson #32

by JC Spencer

Ever wonder how medical scientists can get something so totally backwards?

A new case study shows that one week after starting on cinnamon supplements a 73-year-old woman developed hepatitis. She was on a high-dose of a statin drug. [*American Journal of Case Reports* 4/15]

It is reported that Daniel Brancheau, M.D., of Providence Hospital and Medical Center in Southfield, Michigan, made the statement: "*There were no other medications the patient was taking that could cause the extent of liver damage, except the cinnamon supplements.*"

The woman's doctors said that cinnamon combined with her high dose of statins induced her hepatitis. Researchers noted that coumarin, found in Cassia and Saigon cinnamon can harm the liver. This appears to be the first report of a person experiencing a toxic effect from cinnamon supplements and statins.

Doctors diagnosed the woman with acute hepatitis and determined that the cinnamon was likely to blame. However, there are errors in this knee-jerk diagnose.

Acute hepatitis is from a virus, not just an infection. Can you eat enough cinnamon in ONE WEEK to obtain a toxic dose of coumarin to harm the liver that quickly?

Statin drugs can lower the immune system and provide an opening for the virus. However, it seems quite unlikely the hepatitis virus came riding in on the cinnamon.

Multiple studies support the dangers of cinnamon. Norwegian researchers, whose work was published in the journal *Food and Chemical Toxicology* concluded that using cinnamon on oatmeal or other cereals just a few times a week can exceed the Tolerable Daily Intake (TDI) of 0.07 mg of coumarin. Yet, the highly toxic drug coumadon (from coumarin) comes in 5 mg doses.

Coumarin levels vary in the four types of cinnamon. Saigon cinnamon is commonly used because it has the most intense flavor with the highest level of coumarin.

Several tests show that a teaspoon of the milder cassia cinnamon varied from 5.8 to 12.1 mg of coumarin.

The University of Mississippi analyzed the coumarin content in the four cinnamons with this conclusion:

Saigon 6.97 g/kg	**Indonesian 2.15 g/kg**
Cassia 0.31 g/kg	**Ceylon 0.017 g/kg**

This converts to coumarin parts per million (ppm) with Saigon showing ~7,000 ppm compared to Ceylon ~17 ppm. **Ceylon is the ONLY cinnamon that qualifies for T/C+.**

Smart Sugar Lesson #19 published May 2011 stated. "*All cinnamon is not the same. European health agencies have warned against consuming high amounts of cassia bark, one of the four species of cinnamon, because of its coumarin content. Recent European studies have shown that cinnamon derived from the cassia plant contains this toxic compound, which in large concentrations, is known to cause liver and kidney damage...*"

Smart Sugar Lesson #16 published earlier in 2011 reported, "*Trehalose/Cinnamon can change your life and is one of the most healthful spices in your kitchen. But, caution [about other cinnamon] because Ceylon cinnamon is the only true cinnamon. ... Combine Ceylon cinnamon with the sugar Trehalose and you have two amazing ingredients for your health's future. Besides that, T/C [now T/C+] is so delicious that you will want to sprinkle it on your toast, put it in your coffee or tea, on your salads and desserts.*"

Sources and References
What is T/C+? http://www.endowmentmed.org/content/view/1164
Smart Sugar Lesson #19 http://www.endowmentmed.org/content/view/1168/1/
Smart Sugar Lesson #16 http://www.endowmentmed.org/content/view/1163/1/
http://amjcaserep.com/download/index/idArt/892804
University of Mississippi - Source of Coumarin in Cinnamon
http://www.cinnamonvogue.com/DOWNLOADS/Cinnamon_and_coumarin.pdf
http://www.naturalhealth365.com/food_news/cinnamon_alert.html
http://www.digitaljournal.com/article/323339
http://www.newsmax.com/Health/Health-News/cinnamon-statin-cholesterol/2015/05/15/id/644864/#ixzz3aQIDBkIm
http://www.livescience.com/50838-cinnamon-supplements-statins-liver-risks.html
www.GlycoscienceNEWS.com www.Glycosciencewhitepaper.com
SMART SUGARS www.OneSmartSugar.com/video.html
Expand Your Mind - Improve Your Brain
http://www.endowmentmed.org/ExpandYourMind/MindEbook3.html
Change Your Sugar, Change Your Life http://DiabeticHope.com
Glycoscience Lesson #32 http://www.GlycoscienceNEWS.com/pdf/Lesson32.pdf
http://EzineArticles.com/?expert=JC_Spencer
© The Endowment for Medical Research, Inc. www.endowmentmed.org

From the Home Page of http://endowmentmed.org thousands of our readers have read our Lesson and Article Topics within the Sugar Science Forum:

Smart Sugar Lesson Series

Appreciated Personalities

Clinical Trials Grow in Importance

Missing Sugar Causes Brain Starvation - Triggers Alzheimer's

Huntington's Disease

Toxins and Glycomicscience

Glycomics Humor - glyCOMICS with a point

Training in Reducing Healthcare Costs

Simple Ways To Improve Health

Sciences Supporting Glycomics

Glycomics and Genonmics - the New Healthcare

Trehalose

Trehalose in the NEWS

Using Trehalose - Recipes and Results

Science Papers

Bag Sugars and Sweeteners

Brain Function

Quantum Glycobiology

All topics are accessible from the top of our Home Page at
http://endowmentmed.org or http://forum.endowmentmed.org/index.php

You may wish to explore http://GlycoscienceNEWS.com

Readers have access to hundreds of hours of FREE online materials in the form of articles, reports, and video clips. This is a part of the educational effort of The Endowment for Medical Research.

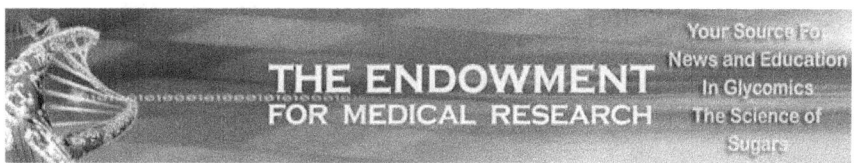

http://endowmentmed.org

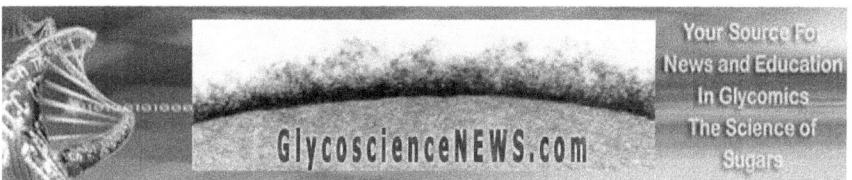

http://GlycoscienceNEWS.com

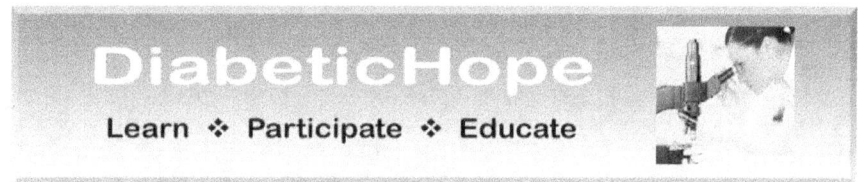

http://DiabeticHope.com

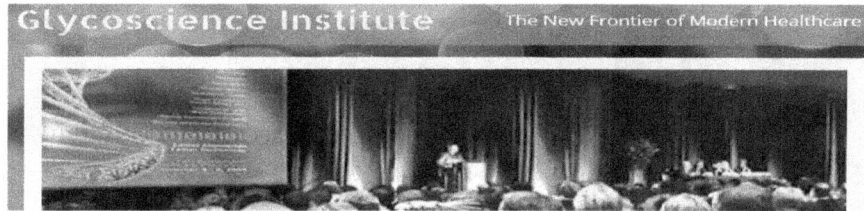

http://GlycoScienceInstitute.com

Short Neurological Tests

Interesting games to self evaluate how well your brain is functioning.

How long does it take you to find the C?

OOOOOOOOOOOOOOOOOOOOOOOOOOOOOOOOOOOOOOOOOOO
OOOOOOOOOOOOOOOOOOOOOOOOOOOOOOOOOOOOOOOOOOO
OOOOOOOOOOOOOOOOOOOOOOOOOOOOOOOOOOOOOOOOOOO
OOOOOOOOOOOOOOOOOOOOOOOOOOOOOOOOOOOOOOOOOOO
OOOOOOOOOOOOOOOOOOOOOOOOOOOOOOOOOOOOOOOOOOO
OOOOOOOOOOOOOOOOOOOOOOOOOOOOOOOOOOOOOOOOOOO
OOOOOOOOOOOOOOOOOOOOOOOOOOOOOOOOOOOOOOOOOOO
OOOOOOOOOOOOOOOOOOOOOOOOOOOOOOCOOOOOOOOOOOO
OOOOOOOOOOOOOOOOOOOOOOOOOOOOOOOOOOOOOOOOOOO
OOOOOOOOOOOOOOOOOOOOOOOOOOOOOOOOOOOOOOOOOOO
OOOOOOOOOOOOOOOOOOOOOOOOOOOOOOOOOOOOOOOOOOO
OOOOOOOOOOOOOOOOOOOOOOOOOOOOOOOOOOOOOOOOOOO
OOOOOOOOOOOOOOOOOOOOOOOOOOOOOOOOOOOOOOOOOOO
OOOOOOOOOOOOOOOOOOOOOOOOOOOOOOOOOOOOOOOOOOO
OOOOOOOOOOOOOOOOOOOOOOOOOOOOOOOOOOOOOOOOOOO
OOOOOOOOOOOOOOOOOOOOOOOOOOOOOOOOOOOOOOOOOOO
OOOOOOOOOOOOOOOOOOOOOOOOOOOOOOOOOOOOOOOOOOO
OOOOOOOOOOOOOOOOOOOOOOOOOOOOOOOOOOOOOOOOOOO
OOOOOOOOOOOOOOOOOOOOOOOOOOOOOOOOOOOOOOOOOOO
OOOOOOOOOOOOOOOOOOOOOOOOOOOOOOOOOOOOOOOOOOO
OOOOOOOOOOOOOOOOOOOOOOOOOOOOOOOOOOOOOOOOOOO
OOOOOOOOOOOOOOOOOOOOOOOOOOOOOOOOOOOOOOOOOOO
OOOOOOOOOOOOOOOOOOOOOOOOOOOOOOOOOOOOOOOOOOO
OOOOOOOOOOOOOOOOOOOOOOOOOOOOOOOOOOOOOOOOOOO
OOOOOOOOOOOOOOOOOOOOOOOOOOOOOOOOOOOOOOOOOOO
OOOOOOOOOOOOOOOOOOOOOOOOOOOOOOOOOOOOOOOOOOO
OOOOOOOOOOOOOOOOOOOOOOOOOOOOOOOOOOOOOOOOOOO
OOOOOOOOOOOOOOOOOOOOOOOOOOOOOOOOOOOOOOOOOOO
OOOOOOOOOOOOOOOOOOOOOOOOOOOOOOOOOOOOOOOOOOO
OOOOOOOOOOOOOOOOOOOOOOOOOOOOOOOOOOOOOOOOOOO
OOOOOOOOOOOOOOOOOOOOOOOOOOOOOOOOOOOOOOOOOOO
OOOOOOOOOOOOOOOOOOOOOOOOOOOOOOOOOOOOOOOOOOO
OOOOOOOOOOOOOOOOOOOOOOOOOOOOOOOOOOOOOOOOOOO
OOOOOOOOOOOOOOOOOOOOOOOOOOOOOOOOOOOOOOOOOOO

How long does it take you to find the 6?

```
99999999999999999999999999999999999999999999999999999999999
99999999999999999999999999999999999999999999999999999999999
99999999999999999999999999999999999999999999999999999999999
99999999999999999999999999999999999999999999999999999999999
99999999999999999999999999999999999999999999999999999999999
99999999999999999999999999999999999999999999999999999999999
99999999999999999999999999999999999999999999999999999999999
99999999999999999999999999999999999999999999999999999999999
99999999999999999999999999999999999999999999999999999999999
99999999999999999999999999999999999999999999999999999999999
99999999999999999999999999999999999999999999999999999999999
99999999999999999999999999999999999999999999999999999999999
99999999999999999999999999999999999999999999999999999999999
99999999999999999999999999999999999999999999999999999999999
99999999999999999999999999999999999999999999999999999999999
99999999999999999999999999999999999999999999999999999999999
99999999999999999999999999999999999999999999999999999999999
99999999999999999999999999999999999999999999999999999999999
99999999999999999999999999999999999999999999999999999999999
99999999999999999999999999999999999999999999999999999999999
99999999999999999996999999999999999999999999999999999999999
99999999999999999999999999999999999999999999999999999999999
99999999999999999999999999999999999999999999999999999999999
99999999999999999999999999999999999999999999999999999999999
99999999999999999999999999999999999999999999999999999999999
99999999999999999999999999999999999999999999999999999999999
99999999999999999999999999999999999999999999999999999999999
99999999999999999999999999999999999999999999999999999999999
99999999999999999999999999999999999999999999999999999999999
99999999999999999999999999999999999999999999999999999999999
99999999999999999999999999999999999999999999999999999999999
99999999999999999999999999999999999999999999999999999999999
99999999999999999999999999999999999999999999999999999999999
99999999999999999999999999999999999999999999999999999999999
99999999999999999999999999999999999999999999999999999999999
```

How long does it take you to find the N and W?

```
MMMMMMMMMMMMMMMMMMMMMMMMMMMMMMMMMMMMMMMMMMMMM
MMMMMMMMMMMMMMMMMMMMMMMMMMMMMMMMMMMMMMMMMMMMM
MMMMMMMMMMMMMMMMMMMMMMMMMMMMMMMMMMMMMMMMMMMMM
MMMMMMMMMMMMMMMMMMMMMMMMMMMMMMMMMMMMMMMMMMMMM
MMMMMMMMMMMMMMMMMMMMMMMMMMMMMMMMMMMMMMMMMMMMM
MMMMMMMMMMMMMMMMMMMMMMMMMMMMMMMMMMMMMMMMMMMMM
MMMMMMMMMMMMMMMMMMMMMMMMMMMMMMMMMMMMMMMMMMMMM
MMMMMMMMMMMMMMMMMMMMMMMMMMMMMMMMMMMMMMMMMMMMM
MMMMMMMMMMMMMMMMMMMMMMMMMMMMMMMMMMMMMMMMMMMMM
MMMMMMMMMMMMMMMMMMMMMMMMMMMMMMMMMMMMMMMMMMMMM
MMMMMMMMMMMMMMMMMMMMMMMMMMMMMMMMMMMMMMMMMMMMM
MMMMMMMMMMMMMMMMMMMMMMMMMMMMMMMMMMMMMMMMMMMMM
MNMMMMMMMMMMMMMMMMMMMMMMMMMMMMMMMMMMMMMMMMMMM
MMMMMMMMMMMMMMMMMMMMMMMMMMMMMMMMMMMMMMMMMMMMM
MMMMMMMMMMMMMMMMMMMMMMMMMMMMMMMMMMMMMMMMMMMMM
MMMMMMMMMMMMMMMMMMMMMMMMMMMMMMMMMMMMMMMMMMMMM
MMMMMMMMMMMMMMMMMMMMMMMMMMMMMMMMMMMMMMMMMMMMM
MMMMMMMMMMMMMMMMMMMMMMMMMMMMMMMMMMMMMMMMMMMMM
MMMMMMMMMMMMMMMMMMMMMMMMMMMMMMMMMMMMMMMMMMMMM
MMMMMMMMMMMMMMMMMMMMMMMMMMMMMMMMMMMMMMMMMMMMM
MMMMMMMMMMMMMMMMMMMMMMWMMMMMMMMMMMMMMMMMMMMMM
MMMMMMMMMMMMMMMMMMMMMMMMMMMMMMMMMMMMMMMMMMMMM
MMMMMMMMMMMMMMMMMMMMMMMMMMMMMMMMMMMMMMMMMMMMM
MMMMMMMMMMMMMMMMMMMMMMMMMMMMMMMMMMMMMMMMMMMMM
MMMMMMMMMMMMMMMMMMMMMMMMMMMMMMMMMMMMMMMMMMMMM
MMMMMMMMMMMMMMMMMMMMMMMMMMMMMMMMMMMMMMMMMMMMM
MMMMMMMMMMMMMMMMMMMMMMMMMMMMMMMMMMMMMMMMMMMMM
MMMMMMMMMMMMMMMMMMMMMMMMMMMMMMMMMMMMMMMMMMMMM
MMMMMMMMMMMMMMMMMMMMMMMMMMMMMMMMMMMMMMMMMMMMM
MMMMMMMMMMMMMMMMMMMMMMMMMMMMMMMMMMMMMMMMMMMMM
MMMMMMMMMMMMMMMMMMMMMMMMMMMMMMMMMMMMMMMMMMMMM
MMMMMMMMMMMMMMMMMMMMMMMMMMMMMMMMMMMMMMMMMMMMM
MMMMMMMMMMMMMMMMMMMMMMMMMMMMMMMMMMMMMMMMMMMMM
```

Did you find the C, the 6, the W, and the N?

Good, that indicates that your brain is functioning well. This exercise and other brain exercises are beneficial for stimulating your brain.

Congratulations!

Now, can you raed the fillowing? It is reported that olny 55 plepoe out of 100 can.

I cdnuolt blveiee that I cluod aulaclty uesdnatnrd what I was rdanieg. The phaonmneal pweor of the hmuan mnid, aoccdrnig to a rscheearch at Cmabrigde Uinervtisy, it dseno't mtaetr in what oerdr the ltteres in a word are, the olny iproamtnt tihng is that the frsit and last ltteer be in the rghit pclae. The rset can be a taotl mses and you can still raed it whotuit a pboerlm. This is bcuseae the huamn mnid deos not raed ervey lteter by istlef, but the word as a wlohe. Azanmig huh? Yaeh and I awlyas tghuhot slpeling was ipmorantt!

Progression of some neurodegenerative challenges can be determined by the patient putting the numbers on the face of the clock.

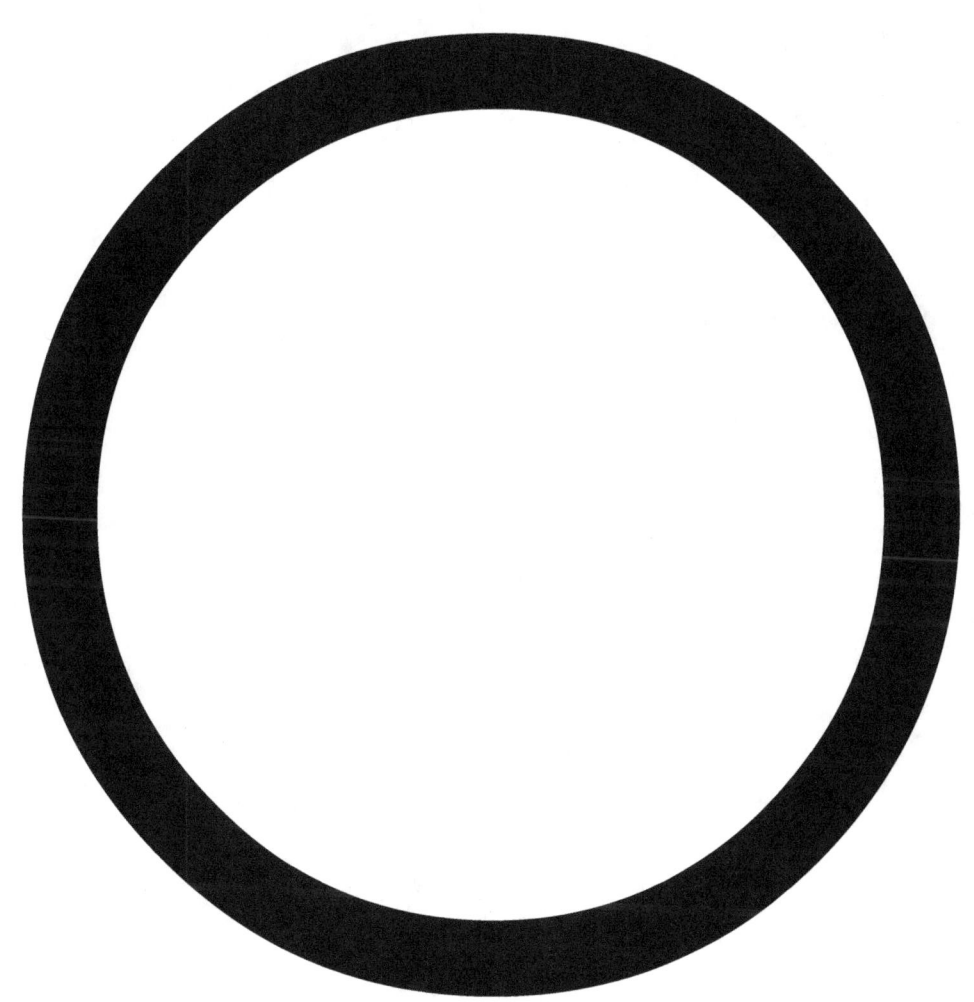

A non evasive diagnostic test for motor skills is for the patient to draw a spiral. Spiral testing is demonstrated on the website of Columbia University at http://cmpl.columbia.edu/diagnostic.html with testing results explained.

Normal

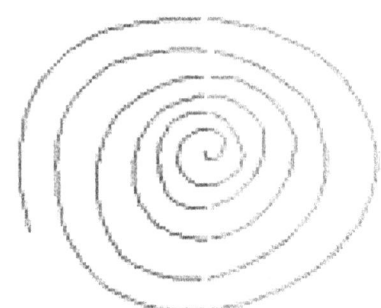

Parkinsons Disease

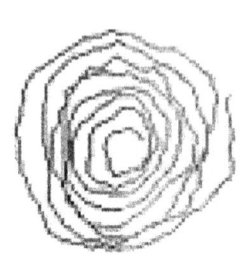

Essential Tremor

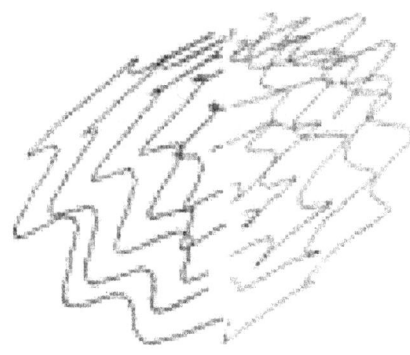

Dystonia

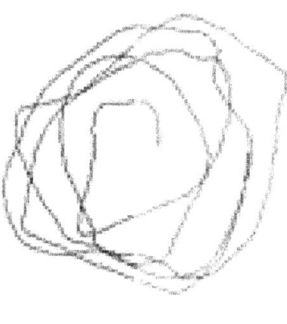

Free educational material for improving brain function is available at
http://endowmentmed.org

THE ENDOWMENT FOR MEDICAL RESEARCH

TRAINING SERIES ORDER FORM

Best way to order is online at http://endowmentmed.org

MAIL ORDER FORM TO: FAX ORDER FORM TO: (281) 397-6789

The Endowment for Medical Research, Inc.
P. O. Box 73089, Houston, Texas 77273   **PHONE US AT:**   (281) 587–2020

Prices subject to change without notice.

Payment accepted in US funds only. Shipped by Flat Rate Priority Mail or Flat Rate Global Priority Mail subject to USPS regulations. If mailing Form, make checks payable to: The Endowment for Medical Research, Inc.

THE ENDOWMENT FOR MEDICAL RESEARCH, INC. IS A 501 (C)(3) NON-PROFIT FAITH BASED SCIENTIFIC RESEARCH, EDUCATIONAL PUBLIC CHARITY.
Non-Profit Tax ID #54-2073489 • DUNS #140133815 for Medical Research and Education Research

14 hours Glycomics DVD Training Series from the First Glycomics Conference for Healthcare Professionals - includes 500 page syllabus	**$199**	**$**
14 hours Glycomics DVD Training Series from First Glycomics Conference for the General Public (does not include 500 page syllabus	**$ 99**	**$**
Old Age Is Not For Sissies with Art Linkletter filmed live as Glycomics Medical Conference Banquet Featured speaker, plus Behind the Scene footage and other interesting and educational footage on 7 tracks. Own this Collector's DVD for a fund raising contribution of $50	**$ 50**	
Stem Cell Survey - A Technical Syllabus on CD Provided for Use by Healthcare Professionals. Evidence that glycomics can increase stem cell proliferation and stem cell function in humans. Learning and Behavior Problems in Children Responsive to Micronutrients Led to Benefits Reported in Infants and Youth and Maternal Alcohol Damage (FAS). Serves as a fund raiser contribution of $50 is shared between The Endowment for Medical Research and the Fisher Institute for Medical Research. **FREE Shipping in USA** Add $20 for all international shipments	**$ 50**	
Visit our Book Store at http://GlycoscienceBooks.com Prices subject to change without notice.		
Orders shipped outside the US subject to custom charges, international shipping costs may vary. Shipments are Flat Rate Priority and Flat Rate Global Priority. For INSURED Express mail information go to http://usps.com. All shipments are FOB Houston, Texas. Payment must be in US Dollars. Contact us at (281) 587-2020 for emergencies.	**Express shipping extra**	
	TOTAL:	**$**

Total includes shipping

Name:_____ Date:_____

Address:_____

City:_____ State/Province:_____ Zip/Postal Code:_____ Country: _____

Home Phone:_____ Business Phone:_____ Cell Phone:_____ Fax:_____

e-mail:_____

☐ Cash ☐ Check #_____ ☐ Credit Card __ Visa __ Master Card __ American Express __ Discover

Credit Card Number: _____ Exp. Date:_____ Code: _____

Name/Address on card (if different from above):_____

City:_____ State/Province:_____ Zip:_____

Signature:_____ Amount Charged: $_____

P.O. Box 73089 Houston, Texas 77273 • 281-587-2020 • FAX 281-397-6789 • info@endowmentmed.org • Website: http://EndowmentMed.org

THE ENDOWMENT FOR MEDICAL RESEARCH, INC. IS A 501 (C)(3) NON-PROFIT FAITH BASED SCIENTIFIC RESEARCH, EDUCATIONAL PUBLIC CHARITY.
Non-Profit Tax ID #54-2073489 • DUNS #140133815 for Medical Research and Education Research   Form Revised 03/01/2016

THE ENDOWMENT FOR MEDICAL RESEARCH, INC.

T/C+ ORDER FORM

Designed to enhance brain function and health

with all the benefits of Trehalose, Ceylon cinnamon and bio-available ionic multi-trace minerals

Designed to help maintain more normal insulin levels which help manage other hormones; optimize blood sugar; slow absorption of carbohydrates and regulate glucose metabolism for maintaining more normal blood sugar levels; keep sugar spikes from happening as fast; slow sugar transport; and help the glycogen process for long term benefit.

Best way to order is online at http://endowmentmed.org or http://E4MR.US

Profits from this sale goes to Medical Research and Education.

MAIL ORDER FORM TO: **FAX ORDER FORM TO:** (281) 397-6789   Ph: 281-587-2020

2 lb Canister T/C+ $77.70 *USA $13.99 s&h*	**$ 91.69**	$
2 - 2 lb Canisters T/C+ $127.70 *USA $13.99 s&h*	**$ 141.69**	$
3 - 2 lb Canisters T/C+ $177.70 *USA $18.99 s&h*	**$ 196.69**	$
Participants in a Six Month T/C+ Pilot Survey $177.70 Receive 2 - 6# Canisters - MUST complete T/C+ Pilot Survey Evaluation Forms or pay full price! *USA $18.99 s&h (all shipped at the same time)*	**$ 196.69**	$
International Orders may be placed online. **Price subject to change without notice.** Orders shipped outside the US subject to custom charges, international shipping costs may vary. Shipments are Flat Rate Priority and INSURED Flat Rate Global Priority. For INSURED Express mail information go to http://usps.com. All shipments are FOB Houston, Texas. Payment must be in US Dollars. Contact us at (281) 587-2020 for emergencies.		$
	TOTAL:	$

The Endowment for Medical Research, Inc.   P. O. Box 73089, Houston, Texas 77273
Ask about larger quantities priced for resale or great savings. Prices subject to change without notice.

Payment accepted in US funds only. Shipped by Flat Rate Priority Mail or Flat Rate Global Priority Mail.
If mailing Form, make checks payable to: The Endowment for Medical Research, Inc.

Name: _____ Date: _____

Address: _____ City: _____ State/Province: _____

Zip/Postal Code: _____ Country: _____ Home Phone: _____

Business Phone: _____ Cell Phone: _____ Fax Number: _____

e-mail: _____

❏ Cash ❏ Check # _____   ❏ Credit Card __ Visa __ Master Card __ American Express __ Discover

Credit Card Number: _____ Exp. Date:_____ Code: _____

Name/Address on card (if different from above): _____

City: _____ State/Province: _____ Zip:_____

Signature: _____ Amount Charged: $_____

P.O. Box 73089 Houston, Texas 77273 • 281-587-2020 • FAX 281-397-6789 • info@endowmentmed.org • Website: http://EndowmentMed.org
THE ENDOWMENT FOR MEDICAL RESEARCH, INC. IS A 501 (C)(3) NON-PROFIT FAITH BASED SCIENTIFIC RESEARCH, EDUCATIONAL PUBLIC CHARITY.
Non-Profit Tax ID #54-2073489 • DUNS #140133815 for Medical Research and Education Research   02/23/2016

THE ENDOWMENT FOR MEDICAL
pH Fusion Tea ORDER FORM

with bio-available ionic multi-trace minerals in a dry phytochemical fulvic acid compound electrostatically blended in sodium. Designed to help human cells achieve a moderately higher pH; have superior nutrient absorption; provide better body hydration; absorb needed ionic multi-trace minerals.

pH Fusion Tea™ is a proprietary nutritional buffer designed to help raise and modulate the human cellular pH level, to lower acid level, and reduce cell stress.

pH Fusion Tea ™ is designed to offset acid overload without interrupting good digestion. The buffer formulation is designed to fortify the cell membrane and to equip the cell for superior nutrient absorption.

Best way to order is online at http://endowmentmed.org or http://E4MR.US

Profits from this sale goes to The Endowment for Medical Research, Inc.

MAIL ORDER FORM TO: **FAX ORDER FORM TO:** (281) 397-6789 • Ph: 281-587-2020
The Endowment for Medical Research, Inc.   P. O. Box 73089, Houston, Texas 77273
Ask about larger quantities priced for resale or great savings.   **Prices subject to change without notice.**

2 lb Trehalose pH Fusion Tea $77.70 *USA $13.99 s&h (2 lb container)*	**$ 91.69**	$
2 - 2 lb Trehalose pH Fusion Tea $127.70 *USA $13.99 s&h (2 - 2 lb containers)*	**$ 141.69**	$
3 - 2 lb Trehalose pH Fusion Tea $177.70 *USA $18.99 s&h (3 - 2 lb containers)*	**$ 196.69**	$
Participants in a Six Month pH Fusion Tea Pilot Survey $177.70 Receives 6 - 2# Canisters - MUST complete Special pH Fusion Tea Evaluation Forms *USA $37.98 s&h (shipped in 2 boxes)*	**$ 215.68**	$
International Orders may be placed online. **Prices are subject to change without notice.** Orders shipped outside the US subject to custom charges, international shipping costs may vary. Shipments are Flat Rate Priority and INSURED Flat Rate Global Priority. For INSURED Express mail information go to http://usps.com. All shipments are FOB Houston, Texas. Payment must be in US Dollars. Contact us at (281) 587-2020 for emergencies.	**TOTAL:**	$ $

Payment accepted in US funds only. Shipped by Flat Rate Priority Mail or Flat Rate Global Priority Mail.
If mailing Form, make checks payable to: The Endowment for Medical Research, Inc.
See http://pHmarker.com for Trehalose Handbook.

Name: _____ Date: _____
Address: _____ City: _____ State/Province: _____
Zip/Postal Code: _____ Country: _____ Home Phone: _____
Business Phone: _____ Cell Phone: _____ Fax Number: _____
e-mail: _____
❏ Cash ❏ Check # _____ ❏ Credit Card __ Visa __Master Card __American Express __Discover
Credit Card Number: _____ Exp. Date:_____ Code: _____
Name/Address on card (if different from above): _____
City: _____ State/Province: _____ Zip:_____
Signature: _____ Amount Charged: $_____

P.O. Box 73089 Houston, Texas 77273 • 281-587-2020 • FAX 281-397-6789 • info@endowmentmed.org • Website: http://EndowmentMed.org
THE ENDOWMENT FOR MEDICAL RESEARCH, INC. IS A 501 (C)(3) NON-PROFIT FAITH BASED SCIENTIFIC RESEARCH, EDUCATIONAL PUBLIC CHARITY.
Non-Profit Tax ID #54-2073489 • DUNS #140133815 for Medical Research and Education Research   03/02/2016

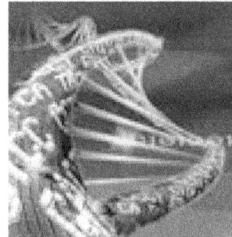

THE ENDOWMENT
FOR MEDICAL RESEARCH

Your Source For News and Education In Glycomics The Science of Sugars

The Endowment for Medical Research is giving birth to the GLYCOSCIENCE INSTITUTE to provide important education and training to physicians and healthcare professionals so their patients can live longer healthier lives. It's becoming more common for modern healthcare professionals to focus on wellness instead of attempting to overcome sickness by treating symptoms. This axiom places the GLYCOSCIENCE EDUCATION AND TRAINING service in high demand. Learn about updates at http://GlycoScienceInstitute.com

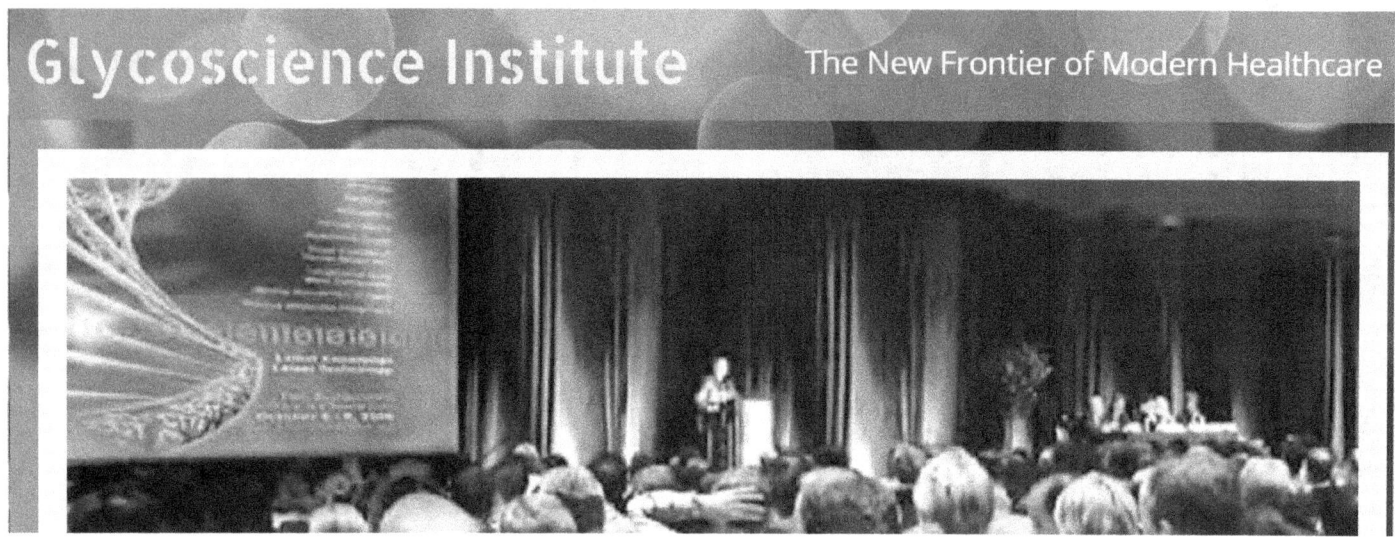

Glycoscience Institute — The New Frontier of Modern Healthcare

About the Author

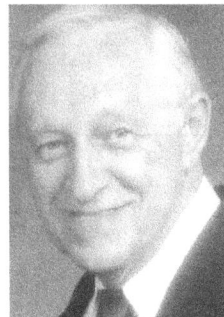

JC Spencer makes practical application of his knowledge of Glycoscience that he has gained during the last two decades. You need not understand the science to Enjoy Smart Sugars and reap their health benefits. The layperson and seasoned medical scientists, professors, and researchers are introduced to new information about this emerging discipline of Glycoscience. Everything points to accelerated and expanded glycan and glycoprotein research, and rightfully so.

He is CEO of The Endowment for Medical Research, Inc, a 501(c)(3) non-profit faith-based medical research and education public charity and think tank based in Houston, Texas, which conducts nutritional surveys throughout the United States, Canada, and some foreign countries. He is also co-founder if the GlycoSience Institute, Inc., a Texas Educational Corporation organized for the express purpose of Glycoscience Education.

For details on booking the author for lectures at universities and fund raising events
contact him at jcs@endowmentmed.org